BIOTERRORISM

How to Survive
the 25 Most Dangerous
Biological Weapons

Pamela Weintraub

Foreword by Paul Rega, M.D.

CITADEL PRESS
KENSINGTON PUBLISHING CORP.
www.kensingtonbooks.com

This book presents information based upon the research and personal experiences of the authors. It is not intended to be a substitute for a professional consultation with a physician or other health-care provider. Neither the publisher nor the authors can be held responsible for any adverse effects or consequences resulting from the use of any of the information in this book. They also cannot be held responsible for any errors or omissions in the book. If you have a condition that requires medical advice, the publisher and authors urge you to consult a competent health-care professional.

CITADEL PRESS BOOKS are published by

Kensington Publishing Corp.
850 Third Avenue
New York, NY 10022

First printing: February 2002

10   9   8   7   6   5   4   3   2   1

Printed in the United States of America

Library of Congress Control Number: 2002100359

ISBN: 0-8065-2398-0

For the first responders, professional and civilian, of 9/11.

CONTENTS

Foreword by Paul Rega, M.D.   ix

Acknowledgments   xiii

Introduction Dark Winter: Defining the Threat   1

THE BACTERIA

1. Anthrax   11
2. Plague   28
3. Tularemia   39
4. Cholera   50
5. Q Fever   57
6. Brucellosis   64
7. Glanders and Melioidosis   70

THE VIRUSES

8. Smallpox   79
9. The Viral Hemorrhagic Fevers   94
   Ebola, Marburg, Lassa, Junin, Yellow Fever, Dengue,
   Rift Valley Fever, Crimean-Congo Fever, and Hantavirus

10. The Equine Encephalitides   114
    Venezuelan Encephalitis (VEE), Western Encephalitis
    (WEE), and Eastern Encephalitis (EEE)

THE TOXINS _____

11. Botulism   123
12. Yellow Rain (T-2 Mycotoxin)   135
13. Staphlococcal Enterotoxin B   145
14. Ricin   149

    Conclusion Family Preparedness   156
    Resources
    A. Characteristics of Biological Agents   187
    B. Cross-Reference of Biological Agents   190
    C. Victim Instruction Form   193
    D. Lexicon of Biological Terror   196
    E. Contact in Case of Emergency   202
    F. Decontamination, Precaution, Sanitation,
       Quarantine: The Supplies   210
    G. Medications and Therapies   215
    References   223

F O R E W O R D

History has shown that the first responders to a disaster, whatever the size, whatever the cause, have not been paramedics or police or firefighters. The true first responders have been the public, the private citizens—family, friends, passers-by. No matter the nationality, the socioeconomic status, or the culture, these people put their own lives on hold and in jeopardy to assist their fellow man. Whether it's a tsunami invading Japan, a hurricane ravaging Key West, or a bombing in Northern Ireland, the average citizen is first on the scene to provide assistance and solace.

We Americans have seen this phenomenon time and time again in our own country. The media have performed a thorough job in emphasizing the heroism of the average citizen. Yet how many more lives could have been saved or further damage prevented had these rescuers received a basic education in disaster first aid? How many fewer injuries would these rescuers have sustained had they been trained in disaster preparedness? Example: A little-known incident occurred after the Oklahoma City bombing when a hospital employee sustained mortal head injuries from a piece of fallen masonry as she was attending a victim. Another example: During a 1995 sarin nerve gas attack in Japan, many of the victims were not those directly exposed to the poison on the subway, but were hospital employees without proper protective gear who received secondary exposure from the victims they were treating.

The federal agencies responsible for the National Emergency Response Plan need to develop a clear, concise, comprehensive Basic Disaster Preparedness and Response course for the American public— the true first responders. The events of September 11 and the subsequent anthrax incidents increase the sense of urgency for the establishment of this concept. The average American has now become a target, and there is no assurance that this will end soon. The key to this new reality is that, although we must accept the fact that we are targets, we must eliminate the notion that we are victims. In keeping with President Bush's idea, each and every one of us must believe that we are the frontline foot soldiers in the defense of our homeland.

To be effective defenders and responders, the American citizen must receive a basic level of disaster training with specific attention to terrorism. Courses do exist for the public, but there is no standardization or requirements or accountability. In addition, there are no incentives. An official national course developed by accepted experts for which tax credits are granted or insurance discounts proffered for successful completion could result in the education of millions of Americans.

This education is especially needed for key issues associated with bioterror. The federal system has expended billions for education, preparedness, and response with regard to biological terrorism, and yet the medical infrastructure is still struggling to meet the challenge of a major bioweapons attack. Hospitals are unable to handle a sudden patient surge. Most health care providers would have difficulty reciting the cardinal features of botulism, let alone prescribing therapy. The legal system must confront a number of conflicting concepts such as societal issues associated with mass quarantine and personal civil liberties.

In this setting, the educated American citizen, the trained American foot soldier, is an essential element and should be a welcomed partner with the American infrastructure in homeland defense. Anything less than this could trigger confusion, increase harm, ensure panic, and improve the terrorist's chance for victory.

This book is a significant advance in the endeavor to improve the knowledge base for all Americans with regard to bioterrorism preparedness and response. A cursory review might cause one to believe that the material is too much for the average reader. With that viewpoint I most heartily disagree. During the first few days when a bioterror hell breaks out, when the local infrastructure is isolated and in disarray, when federal assets are delayed, and when each individual can only depend on one another, it is critical to have as much information as possible. Ms. Weintraub has spent an exhaustive amount of time researching and writing this book. Her sources are impeccable. She fully understands that each person should have some knowledge of the pathophysiology, diagnosis, treatment, and key concepts associated with the major biological weapons because it is conceivable that in a worst-case scenario the immediate medical infrastructure may not have this information.

Perhaps a scenario could better illustrate this. Patient One arrives back in his community from an out-of-state convention. He is accompanied to the local ER by a fellow traveler. His complaints center around a blurring of vision, a slight difficulty in speaking and swallowing, and a perception of generalized weakness. The doctor's basic history-taking and cursory examination fail to elicit any particular finding and the patient is sent home with reassurance. Twenty-four hours later, the patient is admitted to the hospital as a "possible stroke" because of drooping eyelids, slurred speech, and weakness of the arms. Now the friend starts to complain of blurring vision.

Scenario two involves the same patient and complaint. However, now the friend is an educated advocate for his friend. "Doctor, are you sure it's nothing?" "Could it be something else?" "Did you know we were just at a controversial political convention?" "Botulism can start something like this. We're within the incubation period." "I know of at least ten people who were at the same convention. I can find out from them if they are having any problems." "Can you check with the Health Department at the convention site and see what they've heard?" "Doctor, I've just called my colleagues and four of them are having a hard time seeing, two are slurring their words, and one's eyelids are drooping. I think you need to notify our Health Department."

For the first scenario, the correct diagnosis would have been made in 2 or 3 days. However, that delay translates into a delay not only of diagnosis and treatment, but in the critical activation of public health, FBI, and CDC. This delay will feed the media frenzy, increase confusion and fear, and impede the terrorist's capture.

However, the responsibility of each American does not stop with merely reading this book. The successful response to a terrorist attack begins at the community level. Find out whether your hospitals have added an antiterrorist annex to their disaster plans. Do they have a decontamination area and how many victims can be deconned in what span of time? Are there plans to identify and stock ancillary treatment areas to manage an overflow of patients? Is there a stockpile of extra drugs and antidotes for treatment and prophylaxis? Is there a central agency to accumulate and interpret, on a daily basis, data about the general health of the community? Has the medical infrastructure developed courses on weapons of mass destruction and seminars for local health care providers? Have drills been developed specifically dealing with a radiological, chemical, or biological attack? The public should ask these and more questions of their local authorities. It's their right and obligation.

Over the course of the past decade, local, state, and federal authorities have done much to prepare this country for a terrorist attack. The events of this past fall have demonstrated that more still needs to be done. However, any future endeavor cannot be completely successful without the education and participation of the American public. Ms. Weintraub's work will help in achieving that success.

Paul Rega, M.D., F.A.C.E.P.
Medical Program Manager
University of Findlay
Center for Terrorism Preparedness

ACKNOWLEDGMENTS

My greatest debt goes to Dr. Paul Rega, Medical Program Manager, University of Findlay, Center for Terrorism Preparedness and author of *Bio-Terry: A Stat Manual to Identify and Treat Diseases of Biological Terrorism,* now in use at Emergency Departments around the world. In reviewing this manuscript, Dr. Rega provided the benefit of his deep hands-on experience and broad intellectual knowledge to ensure that the information presented would be accurate, sound, and true to the latest that medical research has to offer. In addition, I would like to thank my editor, Michaela Hamilton; my literary agent, Wendy Lipkind; and my husband, Mark, for enduring long talks on the topic of biological terrorism and for asking endless questions, until the terrain I needed to cover in this book crystalized and became clear.

BIOTERRORISM

INTRODUCTION
Dark Winter: Defining the Threat

On September 11, 2001, hours after New York's twin towers crumbled to the ground in the worst terrorist attack in history, the state's Department of Health and the national Centers for Disease Control and Prevention (CDC) were on the scene sampling the rubble and the air. While officials expressed concern over exposure to asbestos, acidic gas, and other contaminated dust and debris, their greater worry was something else—the possibility that the crashing planes had discharged weaponized versions of anthrax, smallpox, or plague. Investigators were not only relieved to find this worry dispelled, but actually surprised.

Three weeks later, with lower Manhattan a war zone, Americans faced a new reality: reservoirs barricaded by police against acts of biological and chemical terror. Crop dusters and hazardous waste trucks, allegedly targeted by terrorists for delivery of killer cargo, were placed under 24-hour surveillance.

But the precautions could not prevent another wave of terror: an anthrax attack in which the U.S. mail would be used to send the deadly bacteria to media celebrities and senators, infecting and even killing staff members, postal workers, and ordinary citizens instead. Gripping the nation in a widening circle of fear in the wake of 9/11, the anthrax letters, as they have come to be known, served to underline our vulnerability without the scale of a true catastrophic event. Indeed, despite the deaths and the panic, the anthrax letters were a sideshow to the war on terrorists abroad.

Whether viewed as a deadly test of the system, a sinister terrorist warning, or a twisted prank, the anthrax letters have provided clarity. Before September 11 we were told it would be exceptionally difficult to wage biological war on America. Now, after the anthrax attacks, we know the truth: we are at risk, and the stakes are high.

Mohammed Atta, the terrorist credited with coordinating the September 11 plot and crashing into World Trade Tower One, reportedly had talks the year before with a high-level Iraqi intelligence official. Although United Nations investigators never found the weapons of biological terror in postwar Iraq, experts have long insisted the nation has extensive germ war stockpiles and a research effort fueled by scientists from the Russian biological-weapons complex Biopreparat.

The truth about Biopreparat came out in 1992, after Ken Alibek, deputy chief of the program, defected to the United States. At that time he told the world that the Soviets had manufactured 80 tons of weaponized smallpox, a virus thought to have been eradicated from the face of the earth. Deeply disturbed by his involvement in the effort, Alibek described other germ war stockpiles ready to be deployed. Bacterial weapons in Russia's arsenal of disease included anthrax, plague, tularemia, brucellosis, Q fever, and glanders, he reported. And in addition to smallpox, viral weapons included Venezuelan equine encephalitis and Marburg, a hemorrhagic fever similar to Ebola. Before he left Russia, said Alibek, weaponized versions of Ebola and Japanese encephalitis were in the works.

As if Alibek's accounting were not enough, in February 2001 William Schneider Jr., chairman of the Pentagon's Defense Science Board, warned that Iraq had stockpiled 19,000 pounds of botulinum toxin, with more than one-half of it weaponized. The Russians, according to Schneider, had stockpiled enough anthrax to kill the world's population four times over. What's more, Schneider's group added, barrier to entry is so low it no longer requires a government to enter the game: with an investment of $250,000, four skilled people could produce enough anthrax to bring about a catastrophic event in three weeks.

Donald A. Henderson, former head of the worldwide effort to eradicate smallpox and new director of the Office of Public Health Preparedness, notes that intelligence sources suggest disenfranchised scientists once part of the Soviet war machine are now so desperate for money they have gone to work for rogue states like Iran, Iraq, Libya and North Korea, where they create weaponized smallpox, among other deadly germs.

In the event of attack, say some experts, U.S. civilians would be sitting ducks. Our health care system already operates at 95% capacity, said the Pentagon board, and, as configured, would be unable to accommodate a mass-casualty event. "The biological warfare task force found that this nation does not have an effective, early capability to assess the biowarfare threat and, as a consequence, cannot prevent such a crisis," the board says. "The infrastructure does not exist to execute the desired consequence-management measures."

So palpable was the threat that some 3 months before September 11, experts studying the potential for biological attack held a trial run at Andrews Air Force Base, gateway to Washington, D.C., and home of Air Force One. Sponsored by the Center for Strategic and International Studies, the Johns Hopkins Center for Civilian Biodefense Studies, the ANSER (for Analytical Services, Inc.) Institute for Homeland Security, and the Oklahoma City National Memorial Institute for the Prevention of Terrorism, the senior-level war game simulated release of weaponized smallpox in Oklahoma, Georgia, and Pennsylvania. As participants played out the scenario, they experienced the epidemic spreading from ground zero to a ring of nearby states and, eventually, some 25 states in all. With the exposed population far greater in number than available doses of vaccine, the medical care system overwhelmed, and schools closed nationwide, officials projected 3 million cases of smallpox and some 1 million deaths.

As the Dark Winter simulation played out, the strategic deployment of smallpox devastated the nation—closing interstate commerce, provoking riots, and bringing a reign of martial law. A single attack of a biological weapon, participants concluded, would be far more devastating than the destruction of New York's twin towers, ultimately crippling not just part of a city but all 50 states.

We are vulnerable. "The government currently lacks adequate strategies, plans, and information systems to manage such a crisis," analysts of Dark Winter concluded. "And it will take substantial investment over years for that to change."

Michael Moodes of the Chemical Arms Institute agreed. Today, he said, the best defense against weaponized germs is preventing the terrorists from using them at all. But how likely is that when, as far as the terrorists are concerned, weaponized germs provide enormous bang for the buck? Conventional weapons like bombs and cruise missiles cost $2,000 per square kilometer of destruction, for instance. At $800 and $600 per square kilometer of devastation, respectively, nuclear and chemical weapons are cheaper by far. But weaponized germs wreak havoc for the rock-bottom cost of $1 a kilometer, making them the least expensive means of mass destruction known to man.

While weaponized germs are cheap and relatively simple to deploy, the aftermath of the event would catapult us into a nightmare of the unknown. "Nothing in the realm of natural catastrophes or man-made disasters rivals the complex problems of response that would follow a bioweapon attack," says Donald Henderson. "The consequence of such an attack would be an epidemic and, in this country, we have had little experience in coping with epidemics. In fact, no city has had to deal with a truly serious epidemic accompanied by large numbers of cases and deaths since the 1918 influenza epidemic, more than two generations ago. Besides nuclear weapons," he adds, "the only other weapons with the capacity to take the nation past the 'point of nonrecovery' are the biological ones."

All nations, including the United States, need to strengthen their capacity to cope with the consequences of the use of biological or chemical agents as weapons, advises Dr. Gro Harlem Brundtland, director-general of the World Health Organization, who recently launched a campaign with that goal in mind. Dr. Brundtland told a meeting of health ministers from the Western Hemisphere that proper surveillance and a quick coordinated response are vital if any deliberate uses of agents such as anthrax or smallpox are to be contained before they infect large numbers of people. Highlighting the key role of the Global Outbreak Alert and Response Network, she asserted that "the world has the capacity and experience to detect and control serious disease outbreaks."

But that capacity may not be realized for years. In the here and now, with the reality of the risk still settling in, the American public is alarmingly unprepared. This might be acceptable if, in fact, there were no means of self-defense. Then we might be well advised to live our lives, keep our fingers crossed, and hope for the best. But interviews with top experts and peer-reviewed articles in August publications from the *Journal of the American Medical Association* to the CDC's *Morbidity and Mortality Report* reveal a host of protective and curative tactics that we, as individual civilians and their personal physicians, can take. While our government gears up to deliver a total, society-wide solution, we need not sit by and do nothing. In the face of a health care delivery system still woefully unprepared, we can take steps to protect ourselves.

In the pages that follow you'll find a practical how-to guide for recognizing, eluding, and treating the 25 most feared weapons of biological terror. From methods of self-isolation and decontamination to appropriate dosing for antibiotics and antiviral medications, readers will learn what they must do to stay alive for days, or even weeks, until authorities arrive on the scene.

The information in these pages is based on peer-reviewed literature from the world's most qualified experts, including university scientists and government agencies. The material, neither classified nor a risk to national security, is freely available—intended not for a cult of survivalists, but for those who would minister to the ill in the face of catastrophic events.

It is, of course, an unfortunate outcome of calamity that public supplies and services—not to mention the flow of information—can shut down just when we need them most. That is the unthinkable scenario that has inspired this book. This is a book for the rational private citizen and his or her family—those committed to sustaining ordinary life despite dangers looming ahead. Without being alarmist, without asking the reader to spend much money or alter lifestyle in any way, this handbook nonetheless constitutes a field guide for those in the trenches, which we now understand to be not just foxholes in Afghanistan or Iraq, but our offices, schools, and homes.

Some will object to this book's sensibility—and, despite its meat-and-potatoes style, label it sensational for delivering the information at all. Some will object to the book's premise, contending it flies in the face of the notion that only collective solutions apply. That's what one man was told when, after the World Trade Center crashes, he called a radio talk show to ask how he might protect himself from the biological threat. "It's being addressed by the government," the host, a physician, said. "It's a public health issue, and individuals need not be concerned." In one sense this is true. As a society, our best hope for survival is collective security. We must act to shut the terrorists down, destroying their devastating stockpiles, their hideouts, and their sources of capital. We must create a rapid response system for civilian defense so that any bioweapon making it through the safeguard can be halted at once.

But as our country gears up for its decade-long war against terrorism, it behooves each individual to do what he or she can to protect themselves and those they love. This book does not propose a social or economic solution to the problem, nor does it suggest that civilians take medical care into their own hands. Rather, it constitutes a short-term road map for surviving the first chaotic days and weeks of a biological attack, when public institutions may be crippled or severely overwhelmed, and when access to information may be hampered, at best.

Given the nature of the threat, the strategies in this book hardly guarantee survival. But all things being equal, they will confer an edge in the face of weaponized germs that, depending upon the specifics, may kill from 30% to 100% of those exposed. Nothing presented in this book is meant to replace or supersede the specific instructions or ministrations of personal physicians, medical professionals, or the health care delivery system. Rather, this information and associated strategies are meant to be used when such resources are unavailable, when the health care system has collapsed, or when the engines of government have been halted or shut down.

This book does not advocate that you stockpile personal supplies of medication, but should that be a strategy you choose to follow, it is important to do so in partnership with your personal physician, not on your own. Remember, antibiotic medications should never be use prophylactically against potential bacterial bioweapons, unless you have evidence there's been an attack, and that you, personally, have been exposed.

One reason for such caution is the threat of smallpox, a virus which, unlike bacterial infections, does not respond to antibiotics. While antibiotics are indeed called for in the event of secondary bacterial infections that sometimes accompany smallpox, they can also, if used indiscriminately, serve to render those infections resistant to treatment. Therefore, while you may indeed possess small, personal quantities of some medications, you must also resist the temptation to do anything with them unless there is an absolute medical need.

We hope our government and medical delivery systems are so organized that they arrive on the scene with antibiotics, vaccines, antidotes—whatever is required—within hours of a bioterrorist attack, and that they have enough information and supplies to service everyone in need. If that occurs, you should consider the suggestions here as merely supplementary, and accept the greater expertise and undoubtedly superior therapies and solutions offered by the Centers for Disease Control and Prevention, the Federal Emergency Management Agency, and your state department of health. But if these officials are late to arrive, if chaos has thwarted their efforts, or if they simply lack sufficient stockpile to service everyone and triage you out of the rescue effort, the information here may help.

THE BACTERIA

Bacteria are single-celled organisms varying in shape and size. They may be spherical (cocci), rod-shaped (bacilli), or even coiled (spirochetes). The shape of each bacterial cell is determined by the structure of its rigid cell wall. The inside of the cell contains genes, made up of DNA, and various organelles required to fuel the life of the bacterium. Many bacteria also have specialized adhesion proteins on their outer surfaces that help them attach to and infect tissue in the host. Under special circumstances some types of bacteria can transform into spores. The spore of the bacterial cell is more resistant to cold, heat, drying, chemicals, and radiation than the living bacterium itself. Like the seeds of plants, spores are a dormant life form, able to germinate and start growing and reproducing when conditions are right.

Bacteria generally cause disease through one of two mechanisms: invading host tissues, and producing poisons, known as toxins. Many disease-causing bacteria use both mechanisms. The diseases they produce often respond to specific therapy with antibiotics. Depending upon the bacteria, a variety of antibiotics over a range of time periods may work best.

In the first section of this book, we cover bacteria as well as rickettsiae—organisms smaller than bacteria, and notable for their inability to live outside of a host. Like bacteria, rickettsiae respond to treatment with antibiotics.

1
Anthrax

Delivery: Contact with skin or inhalation of aerosols.

Symptoms: Two-stage illness begins as flu and progresses, within 36 hours of first symptom, to high-grade infection characterized by fever, profuse sweating, respiratory distress, cyanosis (bluish discoloring of the skin suggesting lack of oxygen), shock, and death.

Timeline: Symptoms in form of flulike illness begin 1–10 days after inhalation. Some 36 hours thereafter, severe illness includes chest pain, respiratory failure, shock, and death.

Can be mistaken for: Tularemia and bartonella (cat scratch fever) as well as many other biological weapons that first present like flu, including the plague, Q fever, and brucellosis.

Treatment: The medications of choice are ciprofloxacin and doxycycline. For severe symptoms, antibiotic cocktails involving two and often three medications work best.

Anthrax in Nature

Anthrax, the disease, has been with us since the dawn of agriculture. It was described in *Exodus* as the fifth and sixth plagues of Egypt, with number five a "grievous murrain" that killed cattle and number six "a boil breaking forth with blains upon man and upon beast throughout the land." Anthrax was later depicted by Virgil in the great poem, *Georgics,*

in 29 B.C. as an agricultural epidemic so hideous "the very stalls" became "carrion-heaps that rot," sheep were "gnawed through and through
with foul disease," and not even the farmer was spared. "Red blisters
and an unclean sweat o'erran his noisome limbs," Virgil wrote of one
poor man.

Anthrax stayed with us even when we moved from the farms to the
factories. In the mid-1800s, mill workers in England sometimes contracted the lethal illness called "woolsorter's disease." Their plight was
the same as that of mill workers in Austria and Germany, where "rag-
picker's disease" afflicted those exposed to fibers, often imported from
abroad.

Caused by the bacterium, *Bacillus anthracis,* anthrax itself is what
scientists term zoonotic—typically spread from animals to humans.
Anthrax is especially threatening because of its ability to form spores—
sturdy, alternate bacterial life-forms that result when nutrients are low or
conditions become hostile to the organism's survival. Rather than simply
perish, *B. anthracis* converts to spores that can survive for months in the
antibiotic-saturated realm of the human body and for decades (some say
centuries) in venues as diverse as the walls of a subway system and the
dirt along a road. Converting to reproductively viable organisms when
conditions become favorable, the spores can inflict serious disease; when
inhaled, the result is generally fatal unless treatment begins almost at
once. Most anthrax in nature is caused by transmission of *B. anthracis*
spores from the hair of goats, sheep, cattle, horses, and swine.

Those who merely touch anthrax spores contract what's known as
cutaneous disease, marked by skin lesions. In fact, *Bacillus anthracis*
derives its name from the Greek word for coal, *anthracites,* because of
its ability to cause black, coallike lesions on the skin. Without treatment,
this form of anthrax kills about 10–20%. Those unlucky enough to *inhale* the spores develop respiratory symptoms, including persistent
cough, which quickly turn into respiratory failure, shock and death.
Called inhalation anthrax, this form of the disease was especially prevalent in the mills of the 19th century, where the new industrial technologies served to aerosolize the spores.

If anthrax was devastating, at least it helped scientists develop theories of disease. It was the first disease for which a microbial origin was
proven—by the founder of the germ theory, Robert Koch, in 1876. It
was also the first disease for which an immunologist named Louis

Pasteur developed a working live vaccine. In his groundbreaking experiment, Pasteur inoculated 25 sheep with a weakened form of the germ. Then he injected those sheep and 25 others with actual anthrax. Only the vaccinated sheep survived.

As the years passed, scientific progress, standards of industrial hygiene and restrictions on imported animal products caused a drastic reduction in natural anthrax. There were only 18 cases of inhalational anthrax in the United States through all the years of the 20th century, most of them in individuals exposed to material processed in textile mills, including goat hair and skin as well as wool. Before the anthrax attacks of 2001, the last U.S. case was recorded in 1976. For almost 25 years, one of the best remaining natural sources of anthrax in the United States were the cattle trails of the Old West, where infected livestock had been left to die. So sturdy were the anthrax spores that they outlived their hosts, surviving in soil for decades, waiting for another "warm body" to amble by.

Anthrax as a Weapon of Biological Terror

With its hardy spores, swift lethality and ease of production, anthrax has loomed as an agent of mass destruction since World War I, when Norway caught a German agent with two vials of anthrax intended for reindeer ferrying allied supplies. When scientists analyzed the Norwegian spores in 1998, they were still alive.

By World War II, almost every country fighting on either side of the conflict had an anthrax program. Indeed, it was Great Britain that demonstrated the killing power of anthrax by using it to kill a flock of sheep on the tiny Scottish Island of Gruinard. The British were so successful that the place called "Anthrax Island" remained contaminated for almost 50 years.

Since those first experiments, anthrax has been stockpiled *en masse* by the superpowers, with the status of an enormous Soviet stockpile still unknown. It has been weaponized by the Iraqis, who produced more than 2,200 gallons of concentrated anthrax bacteria by the end of the Persian Gulf War and admitted loading liquid anthrax into their warheads. It was recovered from the compound of Aum Shinrikyo, the Japanese terrorist cult. And most recently, anthrax was dispatched through the U.S. mail, exposing thousands of American civilians in the aftermath of the World Trade Center attacks on 9/11.

Anthrax's position as a weapon of choice has been bolstered by a series of expert scenarios, each one more apocalyptic than the last: A 1970 World Health Organization (WHO) report concluded that aerosolized anthrax released upwind of 5 million people could lead to 250,000 casualties and 100,000 deaths. That same year WHO conjectured that, under ideal conditions of weather and wind, 50 kilograms of anthrax released from an aircraft along a 2-kilometer (1.2-mile) line could create a lethal cloud of anthrax spores extending some 20 kilometers (12 miles). The aerosol cloud would be colorless, odorless, and invisible following its release. Given the small size of the spores, the Agency added, people indoors would receive the same amount of exposure as people on the street. If the plane let loose near a population center of 500,000, said WHO, you could expect to see 125,000 of those injured and another 95,000 dead. In 1993, the Office of Technology Assessment updated the predictions, estimating that 100 grams of anthrax released to a large American city—in this case Washington, D.C.—could cause between 130,000 and 3 million deaths, depending on the weather and other variables.

The Centers for Disease Control and Prevention (CDC) estimates that a large-scale anthrax attack would carry an economic burden of $26.2 billion per 100,000 people exposed to the spores. But the money would be meaningless compared to the carnage: Ken Alibek, former first deputy director of Biopreparat, the civilian arm of the Soviet biological weapons program, revealed a plan that could have wiped out the population of New York City by loading weapons-grade anthrax into a single warhead, using just a fraction of the total Soviet supply. This sort of attack could kill as many people as a hydrogen bomb.

➤ The scorched Earth scenarios contrast sharply with the slow torture of the anthrax "mail terrorists" striking in the aftermath of 9/11. In a gruesome game of stealth, an assailant managed to strike fear in the heart of America by dispensing anthrax-laced letters to media stars, political figures, and their staffs. From October 4, 2001, to the present time, thousands of people have been exposed to aerosolized *Bacillus anthracis* through the U.S. mail, with missives reaching the halls of Congress and other branches of the government, the major TV networks, and, of course, post offices from Florida to New York.

Though terrifying and tragic, recent anthrax attacks have been limited enough in scope to allow public health officials to move in, diagnosing and treating the sick and the potentially exposed. Even without the specter of social breakdown, our untrained response has engendered some fatal blows. The first victim, a photo editor at the Florida-based tabloid *The Globe,* had the extremely-ill fortune of being the first to enter the medical pipeline. As such, he was unaware that his symptoms might be due to anthrax, and didn't receive the correct treatment until it was too late.

The sixth symptomatic patient, a 47-year-old postal worker at the same mail facility as three previous patients, also gained recognition too late for treatment to help. The man came down with early anthrax symptoms, including nonproductive cough, nausea, vomiting, and stomach cramps on October 16, 2001. Though exposed to anthrax, he was not monitored and didn't think to seek medical attention until October 21, when he reported to the emergency department with vomiting and profuse sweating. Even though his job had placed him at risk, this information was not requested by or clarified for physicians, who rendered a diagnosis of flu, provided intravenous hydration, and sent him home.

When the postal worker returned to the hospital the following day, this time reporting muscle aches, respiratory difficulty, and chills, doctors suspected anthrax and placed him on four antibiotics simultaneously. But his illness was simply too advanced. Increasingly severe respiratory distress required endotracheal intubation and mechanical ventilation. The man died 6 hours after admission to the hospital, and postmortem findings confirmed what had become obvious to all. Blood cultures grew *B. anthracis,* and tissue and serological tests showed evidence of systemic *B. anthracis* infection.

If there is any good news in the terrorist mailings, it is that anthrax, while fatal, may not be as fatal as we thought. While experts previously held inhalational anthrax to be almost 100% fatal after onset of even mild symptoms, we now know antibiotic medication, delivered intravenously and in combination, is curative as long as symptoms have not progressed too far.

Indeed, of the first ten patients to come down with anthrax in 2001, researchers found, eight were in the initial phase of the illness when they sought care. Of these eight, six received antibiotics on the same day, and all six survived. Four patients, including one with meningitis, had full-blown respiratory symptoms when they began antibiotic treatment. All four died.

The anthrax mailings have provoked alarm without precipitating the worst of the nightmare scenarios, but don't be fooled. Remaining dangers were made abundantly clear in 1999, during the congressional testimony of Ken Alibek, who had been responsible for some 32,000 employees and 40 facilities in the former Soviet Union, all devoted to researching agents of biological war. After his defection in 1992, Alibek said, "hundreds of tons of anthrax weapon formulation were stockpiled." Use of anthrax and other weapons "was envisioned on a massive scale, to cause extensive disruption of vital civilian and military activity.

"It is important to note that, in the Soviets' view, the best biological agents were those for which there was no prevention and no cure," Alibek added. So for those agents for which there existed vaccines or treatments, "antibiotic-resistant or immunosuppresive variants were to be developed." This was, in fact, a goal for anthrax, and much effort was put into the development of antibiotic-resistant strains.

Where is all the anthrax stockpiled by our former Cold War adversary? The truth is, no one knows. "Many of Russia's former biological weapons facilities have never been subjected to international inspections or even visits by foreign representatives," Alibek states. Have the stockpiles been sold to the highest bidder? Do they sit in barely guarded storage areas somewhere in the former Soviet Union, tempting quarry for scavengers of biological wares? Such questions may be beside the point, for these days, expertise developed by Soviet scientists is widely available, for free. Indeed, Alibek notes it would be possible to create antibiotic-resistant strains of anthrax just by reading the scientific literature published in Russia in the last few years. "The billions of dollars that the Soviet Union and Russia put into biotechnology research are available to anyone for the cost of a translator," Alibek says.

But all the dire scenarios notwithstanding, could the worst occur? When all the facts are tabulated, the real threat may land somewhere between the stream of poisoned letters and the apocalyptic predictions of the past 20 years.

"Anthrax is only deadly when you inhale a huge number of spores," says nationally recognized anthrax expert, Meryl Nass, M.D., of the Departments of Internal Medicine and Emergency Medicine, Parkview Hospital, Brunswick, Maine. A case in point is the former Soviet city of

Sverdlovsk (now Ekaterinburg), where, in 1979, a faulty filter led to release of anthrax spores from a bioweapons factory. Most experts estimate that no more than 100 people out of more than a million of those
potentially exposed died from anthrax, although the citizens were not
notified of the release, and therefore did not receive prompt antibiotics
or optimal medical therapy.

Anthrax does *not* spread from person to person, Nass points out, and
when it travels with the wind, "it follows a narrow path, and does not
spread out widely over long distances. That is why there were so few
cases in Sverdlovsk. Workers in American factories that were grossly
contaminated with anthrax spores, who inhaled hundreds of spores each
day, almost never developed inhalation anthrax, the most deadly form of
the disease. Therefore, if anthrax is used, it will affect only a limited
area, and relatively small numbers of people. It is a good terrorist
weapon, as any use will strike terror in millions or billions of people.
But it is a *bad* weapon if you are trying to inflict a massive amount of
casualties."

What of the scenario, above, in which 50 kilograms released over,
say, New York City, could kill millions? "You could only achieve massive casualties if you had a plane going back and forth, making multiple
loops over the city, with the wind exactly right," Nass explains. "This
would require that we lose control of the air space over our cities."

Signs and Symptoms

Infection begins after spores are inhaled and deposited in the lungs.
There, the spores germinate into vegetative bacteria, and start to generate toxins that poison the lungs and the rest of the body, rapidly killing
the host. Incubation period from exposure to first symptom is about 10
days. Thereafter, a two-stage illness begins.

In the first, lasting a few hours to a few days, patients come down
with flulike symptoms, including fever, nonproductive cough, vomiting, and malaise. Chest discomfort may be a prominent feature. Some
patients experience a brief improvement or resolution of symptoms before progressing to the second phase, usually within 36 hours of the
time the first stage begins. It is important not to be fooled by this brief
hiatus—comparable to the deceptively still eye of a deadly hurricane, it

has also been called the "anthrax eclipse." For those who are untreated, the eclipse always passes. When it does, about 50% develop hemorrhagic meningitis with headache, stiff neck, and altered mental states. Virtually all suffer high-grade infection characterized by fever, profuse sweating, respiratory distress, and cyanosis (bluish discoloring of the skin suggesting lack of oxygen). And it is lack of oxygen, caused by fluid in the lungs, that brings on the end, often suddenly. Ken Alibek notes that victims of pulmonary anthrax have even been known to die in the middle of a sentence. Of those who are untreated, some 90% succumb.

How Medical Professionals Diagnose Anthrax

Presumptive diagnosis should be made based on signs and symptoms alone, according to the Center for the Study of Bioterrorism and Emerging Infections, St. Louis School of Public Health. There are no readily available rapid and specific tests for early anthrax, but the presumed diagnosis can later by confirmed by culturing bacteria in the blood or by polymerase chain reaction to analyze DNA. Nasal swabs have been used to look for evidence of anthrax, but these may be useless unless performed almost immediately after you have been exposed. Treatment must be initiated as soon as diagnosis is suspected and should not depend in any fashion whatsoever upon a laboratory test. In the event it has been determined that you have been exposed to anthrax in the environment, you will be treated prophylactically.

Care and Treatment

Anthrax must be treated with antibiotics. Antibiotics administered during the incubation period, before symptoms start, dramatically reduce mortality. For victims who have been exposed but lack symptoms, oral antibiotic treatment at home will work.

After symptoms start, experts call for hospitalization, intravenous (IV) antibiotics, and intensive supportive care. Most naturally occurring cases of anthrax are penicillin sensitive, but since it is possible that genetically altered highly resistant strains of anthrax will be encountered during a bioterrorism attack, initial treatment should be empiric until susceptibility testing is available. For those with inhalation anthrax, long-term treatment with multiple antibiotics—up to three or four different drugs, in combination—may be required.

To date, a number of medications have been tested in the lab for efficacy against the disease, and researchers have found that some work better than others:

- Penicillin, for instance, has not been overwhelmingly successful and should be avoided as a single-drug regimen, though it is often successfully added in as the second medicine of a "cocktail" in severe cases.
- Doxycycline is active in vitro and in the animal models, and has been shown especially effective when exposure is by contact with skin. Doxy is considered equivalent to ciprofloxacin with advantages of low price, large stocks, and few side effects.
- Ciprofloxacin (Cipro) is in the fluoroquinolone class of antibiotics, and has been shown to be effective in treatment of animal models of inhalation anthrax, and is FDA approved for this indication. Other fluoroquinolones (levofloxacin, trovaflox-acin, gatifloxacin, and moxifloxacin) are also active in test-tube experiments and would probably be as effective as ciprofloxacin, but have not been tested as thoroughly and have not been FDA approved.
- Clindamycin comes with the possible advantage of stopping protein toxin synthesis, and should be considered if the patient does not respond to Cipro.

Some experts worry that Cipro and doxy may have trouble penetrating the central nervous system (CNS) and passing the blood-brain barrier. They suggest that if victims have evidence of CNS involvement, including brain fog, confusion, or any other neurological symptoms, first-line medications like doxy and Cipro should be used in combination with penicillin or chloramphenicol. Other options for combination therapy are vancomycin and rifampin. Of the fluoroquinolones, gatifloxacin and trovafloxacin probably have the best CNS penetration, and could be considered instead of Cipro.

The latest CDC treatment guidelines follow:

ANTIBIOTICS FOR CUTANEOUS ANTHRAX	
Adults*	Ciprofloxacin 500 mg orally twice a day or doxycycline 100 mg orally twice a day for 100 days.*,**
Children	Ciprofloxacin 10–15 mg/kg every 12 hours or doxycycline in the following dose regimes: 8 years or older and more than 100 pounds: 100 mg orally every 12 hours. Younger than 8 years or less than 100 pounds or both: 2.2 mg/kg orally every 12 hours for 100 days.**,***

* Includes pregnant women and immunosuppressed patients.

** Patients with systemic involvement, extensive edema, or lesions on head or neck require IV therapy and combination therapy (see inhalation anthrax table below).

*** Amoxicillin 500 mg orally three times a day (adults) or 80 mg/kg three times a day (children) can also be used.

Note: Some authorities have expressed concern about use of ciprofloxacin or doxycycline for pregnant women and children since both are inadvisable in pediatric patients and pregnancy. The recommendation is made based on perceived risk/benefit. However, it appears that an acceptable alternative would be to use amoxicillin (500 mg three times a day for adults) for the majority of the 100-day course once the patient has shown clinical improvement.

ANTIBIOTICS FOR INHALATION ANTHRAX		
Patient Category	Initial Therapy: Intravenous***	Long-Term Therapy (Oral)****
Adults*	Doxy 100 mg IV every 12 hours plus 1 or 2 other anitibiotics** or Cipro 400 mg IV every 12 hours plus 1 or 2 other antibiotics.**	Switch to oral therapy when clinically appropriate. Oral therapy can include Cipro 500 mg twice a day or doxy 100 mg twice a day to complete 100 days.
Children	Cipro 10–15 mg/kg IV every 12 hours (maximum 1 gram per day) plus one or two other antibiotics.	Switch to oral antibiotic when clinically appropriate at same dose regimen as at left to complete 100 days.

ANTIBIOTICS FOR INHALATION ANTHRAX		
Patient Category	Initial Therapy: Intravenous***	Long-Term Therapy (Oral)****
	Doxy 100 mg IV every 12 hours plus 1 or 2 other antibiotics** for children older than 8 and weighing more than 100 pounds. Doxy 2.2 mg/kg IV every 12 hours plus 1 or 2 other antibiotics** for those under 100 pounds or less than 8 years of age.	

* Pregnant women and immunocompromised patients should receive the same therapy.

** Other antibiotics that are active in vitro against the current strain: ampicillin, penicillin, clindamycin, clarithromycin, imipenem, vancomycin, rifampin, chloramphenicol.

*** Consider steroids with severe edema or meningitis.

**** One drug may be used when patient has stabilized.

Note: Once patients have stabilized clinically, the IV treatment may be switched to oral, and monotherapy (treatment with a single drug) may be used to complete the 100-day course.

Postexposure Prophylaxis Prophylaxis should be provided to all persons who may have been directly exposed to the initial release. It is critical that antibiotics be administered as soon as possible after potential exposure, before symptoms appear, because this offers the best chance of survival. Patient contacts do not require prophylactic treatment because anthrax is not contagious from person to person:

- Oral antibiotic therapy should be provided for 100 days; this may be reduced if vaccine is administered.
- Ciprofloxacin 500 mg orally twice a day or doxycycline 100 mg orally twice a day.
- Women who are or might be pregnant should use ciprofloxacin, or, if their physicians are concerned about the side effects of this medication, amoxicillin 500 mg orally three times a day. Pregnant women should avoid doxycycline, which may have more potential for adverse fetal and maternal effects.

The CDC's recommendation for two or three types of antibiotic for inhalational anthrax is supported by evidence that bioweaponeers have already created anthrax resistant to common antibiotics, and by findings that anthrax can *develop* antibiotic resistance as treatment proceeds. In December 2001, for instance, Scientists at the 41st Annual Interscience Conference on Antimicrobial Agents and Chemotherapy announced a finding: patients with *Bacillus anthracis* can develop resistance to many of the antibiotics used to treat them over time. The team, headed by Dr. Itzhak Brook of the Armed Forces Radiobiology Research Institute in Bethesda, Maryland, cultured the *B. anthracis* bacteria in different environments using a variety of antibiotics. The group found that bacteria exposed to quinolone antibiotics—the class that includes Cipro—developed resistance to drugs. Other quinolones, including ofloxacin and gatifloxacin, also caused bacteria to develop resistance, but more slowly.

Brook reported that cross-resistance was seen within the quinolone class, but all quinolone-resistant microbes were sensitive to doxycycline. Conversely, a doxycycline-resistant culture was sensitive to Cipro and other quinolones. The team found the bacteria also developed resistance to the macrolide class of antibiotics that includes zithromax, clarithromycin and erythromycin.

The recommendation for a 100-day course of antibiotic treatment emerged only in December 2001. Prior to that experts recommended a 60-day course, based largely on experiments with primates, where researchers found that a 30-day treatment was often followed by late relapse, while 60 days of antibiotic therapy was protective.

More recently, studies suggest spores can survive in the body for up to 100 days. To be on the safe side, experts now recommend 100 days of treatment or 30–60 days of treatment, as long as the patient is vaccinated before the treatment stops.

While the treatment for true cutaneous anthrax is just 10 days, the CDC has changed this to the full regimen advised for inhalational anthrax out of fear that those involved in bioterrorist attacks may, unknowingly, contract both forms of the disease.

The latest addition to the anthrax treatment arsenal, meanwhile, is an immune globulin: an experimental protein culled from blood of soldiers who received anthrax vaccine. This treatment, which experts say could be pushed through approval rapidly in emergency, is an adjunct to antibiotic treatment that works by destroying the anthrax toxin, not the bacteria itself.

The truth is that no one really knows how to treat anthrax infection. We are currently operating at the outer edges of knowledge about a disease with which there is little experience. After all, prior to 2001, there were only 18 cases of inhalational anthrax in the United States in 100 years. Will anthrax spores survive more than 60 days of antibiotic treatment? How about more than 100 days? There is no expert who can reassure those exposed, beyond a doubt, that once antibiotic treatment is stopped a critical mass of *Bacillus anthracis* spores won't activate in the moist caverns of the body, spawning anthrax, the disease.

Vaccine   As with those who have actually contracted anthrax, the disease, those merely exposed to *Bacillus anthracis* spores are being advised, by some, to seek vaccination before the regimen of antibiotics end. Vaccine protocol is as follows:

- Vaccination consists of an initial six-dose series followed by an annual booster. All doses are to be .5 ml subcutaneously.
- Initial series: 0, 2, and 4 weeks after exposure, then 6, 12 and 18 months after exposure.
- Booster doses are required annually to maintain immunity.
- For those who received doses prior to exposure, provide a single booster unless the initial three-dose series was completed within the previous 6 months.

Reflecting its experimental status, the anthrax vaccine was, until December of 2001, approved only for the military, where it was presumed troops might be at risk for exposure to biological weapons of war. But fear that anthrax spores may survive three months or more of antibiotic treatment has caused Tommy G. Thompson, Secretary of Health and Human Services to offer the vaccine to exposed Post Office and Congressional employers out of what he says is "an abundance of caution." So divided are experts on this issue that while Capitol Hill doctor John Eisold, a retired admiral, recommended that Congressional staff be vaccinated, the Post Office told its people to hold off. Apparently getting their cue from the Pentagon, Congressional employees lining up for the vaccine have been told it has few side effects. Postal

workers, who say they would be guinea pigs, point to the roiling controversy the vaccine has caused in the military, where hundreds of personnel have reported permanent, debilitating side effects and have even
endured court marshal rather than accept vaccination, as regulations require they do.

Indeed, skepticism over the vaccine seems to be significant, despite official claims that problems are rare. According to Representative Christopher Shays, a Connecticut Republican who held hearings last year on the
anthrax vaccine, the product may be dangerous because neither it nor the
plant that manufactures it has yet been approved by the FDA.

Meryl Nass, M.D., one of the vaccine's most outspoken critics,
meanwhile, states these dangers are very real. Explaining the argument
she makes in the May, 2002 issue of the *American Journal of Public
Health,* Nass says the problem with the vaccine "is that it is simply not
safe, and the odds of getting sick as a result of vaccination may be
10–35%, based on a considerable amount of anecdotal evidence, including a study from the UK published in 2000 in the *Journal of the Royal
Army Medical Corps,* and five additional studies of the relationship between Gulf War illnesses and vaccination." Nass believes that those who
receive the vaccine will be at risk for developing autoimmune disease
from which they may never recover.

Rather than face the risk of side effects, Nass believes, "those recently exposed to anthrax, who have received 100% effective protection
with antibiotics, can continue this prophylaxis a bit longer, or watch
closely for any signs of infection and receive immediate treatment if this
occurs."

Antibiotic and vaccine treatment for anthrax is today a moving target, and the risk-benefit ratio of all the options has not yet been clarified
for the exposed. The story is still being written as this book goes to
press. If you find that you are faced with this decision, make sure you
have researched all sides of the issue. This is one situation in which the
patient must double as medical consumer watchdog, speaking to his or
her personal physician but also digging deeper, pulling up the latest data
in a decision that may, literally, be a matter of life and death.

Decontamination   The highest risk of infection occurs during the
initial release while a large concentration of anthrax spores remain airborne; in ideal conditions, this is estimated to be up to 1 day. But in fact,
spores are incredibly hardy and may survive for years in soil, resulting

in secondary cases now and then. Given this danger, decontamination of exposed surfaces is essential. But this is not the time for you to rush in with a sponge and a spray bottle of disinfectant. If you suspect spores in or near your home, vacate the premises and call in the government to help with the decontamination task.

As to your own person, remove any clothes directly exposed to anthrax, place them in a plastic bag where they will not be disturbed, and make sure to shower with a washcloth and plenty of soap and shampoo as soon after the incident as possible.

How to Handle Anthrax Letters

In the wake of the recent anthrax attacks, the CDC has issued the following instructions for dealing with the threat of anthrax in the mail.

1. Do not shake or empty the contents of any suspicious envelope or package; do not try to clean up powders or fluids.
2. Place the envelope or package in a plastic bag or some other type of container to prevent leakage of contents.
3. If you have no container, cover the envelope or package with anything (e.g., clothing, paper, trash can) and do not remove this cover.
4. Then leave the room and close the door, or section off the area to prevent others from entering (i.e., keep others away).
5. Wash your hands with soap and water to prevent spreading any powder to your face or skin.
6. If you are at home, report the incident to local police. If you are at work, report the incident to local police, and notify your building security official or an available supervisor.
7. If possible, list all the people who were in the room or area when this suspicious letter or package was recognized. Give this list to both the local public health authorities and law enforcement officials for follow-up investigations and advice.
8. Remove heavily contaminated clothing and place it in a plastic bag that can be sealed; give the bag to law enforcement personnel.
9. Shower with soap and water as soon as possible. Do not use bleach or disinfectant on your skin.

What You Need to Know to Survive
an Attack of Anthrax

- As soon as you suspect that you may have been exposed to anthrax, seek medical help.
- If there is evidence that you may have inhaled or had physical contact with anthrax spores, make sure to start prophylactic treatment at once.
- If physicians question your belief that you have been the victim of an anthrax attack, explain why you are convinced: Are you the CEO of a flag company, a postal worker, or a political intern or aide? If so, explain to emergency department personnel your working environment and the reason why you may have met with foul play. There have been so many hoaxes and so much hysteria surrounding anthrax, it may be necessary to overcome skepticism to make your case.
- Take note that experts have now increased their recommendation for prophylactic treatment with antibiotics from 60 to 100 days unless an individual is vaccinated before treatment stops. The reason is evidence indicating those with high dose exposure may retain enough spores to cause anthrax after the 60-day period is up.
- Because this disease is often fatal, a cavalier attitude toward completing your antibiotic regimen can be deadly, indeed. Make sure the physicians you consult are treating you aggressively enough— and then make sure you take the medication for the full course of treatment, even if it seems excessive or long, and even if you do not feel ill.
- If at all possible, seek treatment from a facility, organization, or individual with experience in dealing with anthrax.
- Unless you receive a nasal swab immediately after exposure, it will be a useless predictor of your potential for infection.
- When developed as a biological weapon, bacteria can have antibiotic resistance genes introduced, rather simply. Since Cipro and doxycycline have been advocated for anthrax since before the Gulf War, an adversary might specifically try to overcome those antibiotics. So it is impossible to know for sure what will work, in advance of an attack. "If there is an anthrax release, the organism will be cultured and we will know within 48 hours what antibiotics to use.

- If you are in the vicinity of an attack, the best protection is to get inside and close all windows and doors. As long as you do not breathe in the tens of thousands or more spores required to induce illness, you should be fine.
- Because you would have to know the exact timing of an anthrax attack for gas mask protection, this device is unlikely to help. But if you must have one, make sure it prevents inhalation of particles greater than one micron in diameter. You can find recommended surgical mask sources in the resource guide at the end of this book. You should seek to buy inexpensive, disposable masks with HEPA filters, but keep in mind that they will not afford you complete protection unless you have them professionally fitted. Call your local hospital to inquire about availability of a fitting in your area.
- You may be asked to either get vaccinated or to extend the length of your antibiotic therapy. The efficacy of various therapeutic strategies is currently a moving target, and you will need to access the latest information, especially the treatment outcomes of those exposed to anthrax through the mail in 2001, to decide what is right for you. The important thing, here, is to use your skills as a medical consumer. Do your own investigation rather than relying on the opinion of any single physician. Weigh all the data, review all the claims and counter claims and, if you are able, go back to read some of the recent literature in the peer-review, referenced at the back of this book. Remember that while some experts say the vaccine only rarely produces side effects, others say it can cause permanent autoimmune disease in a significant percent of the inoculated. Remember, too, that some experts state that 60 or even 100 days of antibiotic treatment may not be enough to stop a case of inhalational anthrax in those who have been exposed—unless they also receive a vaccine.
- Aerosolized anthrax can cause symptoms anywhere from two days to six weeks after exposure, so be vigilant if you think you may have been exposed.
- Report suspected cases of inhalational anthrax to your local health department. The local health department is responsible for notifying the state health department, the FBI, and local law enforcement. The state health department will notify the CDC.

2

Plague

Delivery: Inhalation or ingestion of aerosols; flea bites; direct contact with open skin.

Symptoms: Presents as flulike illness. Accompanied by headache, cough, vomiting, cramps, fever, chills, malaise, and diarrhea. In pneumonic plague, cough (including bloody or rhaspy cough) and chest pain manifest within 24 hours of the first symptoms. In bubonic plague, bacteria are transported to lymph nodes, which become swollen and painful. All forms can progress to shock, multiorgan failure, and death.

Timeline: Symptoms develop from 1 to 6 days following exposure. Without treatment, 90–100% die within 6 days of the first symptom.

Can be mistaken for: Tularemia and bartonella (cat scratch fever).

Treatment: The medications of choice are streptomycin, delivered through intramuscular (IM) route, or gentamicin, via IM or IV. Oral alternatives include doxycycline, chloramphenicol, and ciprofloxacin.

The Plague in Nature

The plague has been a scourge of humanity since biblical times. The book of I Samuel describes a plague that devastated the Philistines after they stole the Ark of the Covenant from the Israelites in 1320 B.C. Their punishment was biblical, indeed: "The Lord's hand was against that city, throwing it into a great panic. He afflicted the people of the city, both young and old, with an outbreak of tumors in the groin." The tumors were likely the buboes, or swellings, we understand to characterize bubonic plague today.

Thereafter, the plague began to make regular appearances in the countries bordering the eastern Mediterranean Sea. In 430 B.C., Sparta won the Peloponnesian War, say historians, partly because of the plague of Athens. And in A.D. 541–542, the first great pandemic of the common era killed as many as 100 million Europeans, including 40% of the population of Constantinople. This first great pandemic is said to have wiped out between 50 and 60% of the human population worldwide.

Smaller epidemics continued to follow this plague until the arrival of the second pandemic, known as the Black Death. Historians now think they can explain why this reign of terror was visited upon Europe. Plague bacteria, they note, probably entered Europe via the trans-Asian silk road during the early 14th century, carried by fleas caught in bales of marmot fur headed for market. When furs were unpacked in Astrakhan and Saray, the fleas, having survived the journey, jumped from casings in search of nourishment most often, blood from a human leg. From there, the plague spread west. It arrived in what is now Ukraine on the Black Sea in 1346, where, historians surmise, it infected the large rat population, part of which stowed away on ships bound for major European ports. By 1348, plague had entered Britain at Weymouth.

The Black Death killed 24 million people between the years 1346 and 1352 and another 20 million by the end of the 14th century. Without antibiotics—or any understanding of bacterial illness at all—populations were defenseless. The plague continued its assault through 1720, with a final stop in Marseilles. From the 15th to the 18th century, 30 to 60% of the people in major cities such as Genoa, Milan, Padua, Lyons, and Venice died of the plague.

The second pandemic eventually subsided. Though no one knows exactly why, factors including the cooler European climate, the use of soap, and the displacement of the black rat, *Rattus rattus,* by the brown rat, *Rattus norvegicus,* likely played a role.

The third, or modern, plague pandemic arose in 1894 in China and spread throughout the world via modern transportation. It arrived in Bombay in 1898, killing some 13 million Indians. And it arrived in the United States in 1900, marked by the discovery of an infected Chinese laborer in the basement of a San Francisco hotel. It thereafter spread north to Washington State and east to New York and New Orleans.

But already progress was being made. It was in 1894 as well that Alexandre J. E. Yersin discovered that *Yersinia pestis,* a bacterium, was the cause of the plague. After general rat control and hygiene measures were instituted in various port cities in 1925, urban plague vanished. The few cases reported since have all been acquired in more rural locales.

The Plague as a Weapon of Biological Terror

The first attempt at biological warfare probably took place at the Crimean port city of Caffa on the Black Sea during the years 1346–1347. There, during the conflict between Christian Genoese sailors and Muslim Tatars, the Tatar army was struck with plague. Turning tragedy to strategy, the Tatar leader is said to have catapulted corpses of Tatar plague victims at the Genoese sailors, who became infected as well.

Modern scientists note that the Genoese probably became infected by a local population of rats, not by the corpses. After all, an infected flea—the primary mode of natural transmission—leaves its host as soon as the corpse cools.

Bioterrorists have come a long way since the 14th century. Modern living conditions, public health, and antibiotics make natural pandemics unlikely, but according to experts, terrorist attacks of weaponized plague pose a serious threat. One danger of even a few cases of the plague is its ability to cause wholesale panic. A çase in point is Surat, India, where, in 1994, just a few infected individuals caused 500,000 to flee a "plague epidemic" that never came.

But weaponized plague is hardly just a scare tactic. Far more lethal than the natural variety, it is an effective agent of death. What's more, it has been under development as a modern biological weapon for some 60 years.

During World War II, at its secret biological warfare research unit in Manchuria, for instance, the Japanese army perfected a means of delivering weaponized plague. Their experiments revealed that just delivering the microbes by bomb would be ineffective, since the heat and high pressure of the explosion killed all the microbes. To get around the problem, they used the human flea, *Pulex irritans*, an organism resistant to air drag, to simultaneously protect the bacteria and target humans. The flea could deliver up to 24,000 plague organisms with a single bite. As a bonus, the Japanese reasoned, the flea could also infect rats, setting the scene for a prolonged epidemic instead of a one-time shot. The group also developed special "clay bombs" that enabled up to 80% of the fleas to survive.

The Japanese used their plague technology on at least three occasions against China during World War II—not by dropping bombs but, rather, by air-dropping a bizarre concoction of plague-infested wheat and rice grains, pieces of paper, cotton wadding, and other unidentified particles. In all three instances, people started dying within a few weeks of the attacks. In this case, no fleas were required; plague can also live in and spread through the environment—ultimately infecting rats and humans—through grains like rice.

In the 1950s and 1960s, the U.S. and Soviet biological weapons programs both developed means of aerosolizing plague particles, making them especially to be inhaled and reach the lungs. More than ten institutes and thousands of scientists were assigned to work with plague in the former Soviet Union, and these researchers and their expertise may still be for sale. According to reports from a defecting Soviet microbiologist, the Soviet Union was successful in its effort to genetically engineer a dry, antibiotic-resistant form of the plague, a goal he said had been one of their top priorities for years.

Experts in bioterrorism consider the plague a serious threat. Not only is it highly fatal and contagious, it is also stored in microbe banks around the world. Furthermore, there are many reports of well-developed technologies for mass production and aerosol dissemination.

A 1970 World Health Organization assessment asserted that, in a worst-case scenario, a dissemination of 50 kg of *Y. pestis* in an aerosol

cloud over a city of 5 million might result in 150,000 cases of pneumonic plague, 80,000–100,000 of which would require hospitalization,
and 36,000 of which would result in death.

Signs and Symptoms

As potentially devastating as the plague may be, it is nonetheless
treatable. For that reason, understanding the epidemiology and the clinical presentation could go a long way toward stanching the damage in
the wake of an attack.

According to the Johns Hopkins Center for Civilian Biodefense
Studies, initial cases would appear in about 1–2 days following the
aerosol cloud exposure, with many people dying quickly after the onset
of symptoms. Human experience and animal studies suggest that the incubation period in this setting is 1 to 6 days. Since there are no effective
advance warning systems and no rapid diagnostic test, the first sign of a
bioterrorist attack would likely be the symptoms themselves.

In almost all cases, the first symptoms of plague appear much like
those of the flu: fever, chills, muscular pain, weakness, and headache.
Also common are gastrointestinal symptoms like nausea, vomiting, diarrhea, and abdominal pain. In pneumonic plague, the most severe form
of the disease and the version that terrorists would bring, chest discomfort, cough, and breathlessness appear within 24 hours of the first symptoms. By days 2–4 of the illness, one can expect a bluish cast to the skin
(caused by lack of oxygen in the blood), respiratory distress, and severe
chest pain. Death, when it comes, is generally the result of overwhelming bacterial infection, DIC (disseminated intravascular coagulopathy)
caused when a malfunction of the clotting mechanism causes abnormal
bleeding, and multiorgan failure.

While pneumonic plague is by far the most dangerous, it is helpful to
be aware of all forms of the disease:

Pneumonic Plague The least common variety, in nature, where it
accounts for less than 14% of cases, this is nonetheless expected to be
the most prevalent presentation in a bioterrorist attack. It is the most
catastrophic form of the disease, characterized by severe pneumonia
acquired via respiratory tract. Clotting abnormalities cause bleeding

from various sites of the body and red or purplish spots and patches on the skin. Blood may clot in the nose, fingers, ears, and toes, leading to gangrene and death of surrounding tissue: accounting for the black extremities often seen in photographs of plague victims. Overall mortality of pneumonic plague without treatment approaches 100%, according to most experts, although some consider it to be somewhat lower.

Bubonic Plague In nature, the most common form of the disease, accounting for between 75 and 97% of all cases. Characterized by painful swellings, called buboes, under the arms and in the groin area. Contracted through the bite of an infected flea or by handling infected animals. Overall mortality rate without antibiotic treatment is 50%. Unlikely to emerge in a bioterrorist setting. Some 25% of those with bubonic plague advance to the more dangerous, septicemic format of the disease, a deadly body-wide infection, described next.

Septicemic Plague Accounts for less than 20% of all cases in nature. Characterized by systemic infection, and said to kill between 22 and 50% of its victims. Symptoms include chills, fever, low blood pressure, vomiting, diarrhea, blood clots, gangrene, and purple and red spots or splotches on the skin.

Six percent of those with plague develop plague meningitis, an infection of the brain.

How the Disease Is Diagnosed by Medical Professionals

There are currently no widely available rapid confirmatory diagnostic tests. A presumptive diagnosis can be made quickly based on symptoms and concurrent lab results, especially if there is a high index of suspicion. Confirmatory tests can be done through blood, sputum (if pneumonic), bubo aspirates (if bubonic), and central spinal fluid (if meningitis occurs). However, waiting for lab results before treating would be a death sentence. Other clues include elevated white blood cell clotting factors and elevated liver enzymes, consistent with multi-organ failure. In addition, the x-ray in pneumonic plague can show patchy or consolidated areas in the chest and lungs.

Care and Treatment

Antibiotics are the treatment of choice—and the only treatment likely to make a difference in the event of a bioterrorist attack with the plague. Rapid treatment is essential, according to St. Louis's Center for the Study of Bioterrorism and Emerging Infections, because half of untreated patients with bubonic plague will die, as will virtually all of those with pneumonic plague. These numbers can be reduced to less than 5% and 20–40%, respectively, if antibiotic therapy starts within 18–24 hours of symptom onset.

For those already infected, says the Center, treatment guidelines will ideally involve intravenous or intramuscular delivery. Optimally, the medical system will be geared up to accommodate all victims' needs. In case of mass casualties, it's possible that most people will have access only to more common oral antibiotics. Infected and exposed individuals alike should follow treatment guidelines until all symptoms are gone and 7 days past the last possible exposure.

Treatment recommendations presented here come from the Working Group on Civilian Biodefense, made up of 25 representatives from major academic medical centers and research, government, military, public health, and emergency management institutions and agencies. These guidelines were printed in the *Journal of the American Medical Association* in May 2000.

In the contained casualty setting, where there are just a few cases, patients should be able to obtain the most effective treatments, as follows:

Adults, Preferred Choices

- Streptomycin, 1 gram IM every 12 hours for 10 days. Caution: This treatment should be avoided by pregnant or lactating women.
- Gentamicin, 5 mg/kg IV or IM once a day every day for 10 days or 2 mg/kg loading dose followed by 1.7 mg/kg IM or IV three times a day for 10 days.

Adults, Alternative Treatments

- Doxycycline, 100 mg IV twice daily or 200 mg IV once daily for 10 days.
- Chloramphenicol, 25 mg/kg IV four times daily for 10 days.
- Ciprofloxacin, 400 mg IV twice daily for 10 days.

Children, Preferred Choices

- Streptomycin, 15 mg/kg IM every 12 hours for 10 days.
- Gentamicin, 2.5 mg/kg IV or IM three times a day every day for 10 days.

Children, Alternative Choices

- Doxycycline, 100 mg IV twice daily for 10 days if weight is greater than 100 pounds; 2.2 mg/kg IV twice daily for 10 days if weight is less than 100 pounds.
- Chloramphenicol, 25 mg/kg IV four times daily for 10 days.
- Ciprofloxacin, 15 mg/kg IV twice daily for 10 days.

Pregnant Women, Preferred Choice

- Gentamicin, 5 mg/kg IV or IM once a day every day for 10 days or 2 mg/kg loading dose followed by 1.7 mg/kg IM or IV three times a day for 10 days. The Working Group notes that gentamicin poses a particularly low risk to the fetus.

Pregnant Women, Alternative Choices

- Ciprofloxacin, 400 mg IV twice daily for 10 days.
- Doxycycline, 100 mg IV twice daily or 200 mg IV once daily for 10 days.

In a mass casualty setting, delivering IV antibiotics to thousands of people in need will be virtually impossible. In that instance, the Working Group recommends the following oral antibiotic protocols for those who are symptomatic as well as those who have been exposed and are in need of prophylactic treatment:

Adults, Preferred Choices

- Ciprofloxacin, 500 mg every 12 hours for 10 days.
- Doxycycline, 100 mg every 12 hours for 10 days.

Adults, Alternative Choice

- Chloramphenicol, 25 mg/kg orally four times daily for 10 days. (Oral version of this medication unavailable in the United States.)

Children, Preferred Choices

- Ciprofloxacin, 20 mg/kg orally every 12 hours for 10 days.
- Doxycycline, 100 mg every 12 hours for 10 days if more than 100 pounds. If less than 100 pounds, 2.2 mg/kg orally twice daily.

Children, Alternative Choice

- Chloramphenicol, 25 mg/kg orally four times daily for 10 days. (Oral version of this medication unavailable in the United States.)

Pregnant Women, Preferred Choices

- Ciprofloxacin, 500 mg every 12 hours for 10 days.
- Doxycycline, 100 mg every 12 hours for 10 days.

Pregnant Women, Alternative Choice

- Chloramphenicol, 25 mg/kg orally four times daily for 10 days. (Oral version of this medication unavailable in the United States.)

In addition to antibiotic treatment, people with established ongoing exposure to a patient with pneumonic plague should wear simple masks and should have patients do the same. Patients should be isolated from others until they have been on antibiotic therapy for 48 hours.

What You Need to Know to Survive an Attack of the Plague

- There is no widely available rapid diagnostic laboratory test for the disease.
- The plague is highly contagious from person to person. Once an epidemic has begun in your area, you should seek treatment whether you are symptomatic or not.
- People with household or face-to-face contacts with known plague victims should continue prophylactic treatment for 7 days following the last exposure.
- If you are caring for a loved one, make sure to wear a surgical face mask, surgical gloves, and other protective gear.
- Isolate the stricken from the rest of the family; if possible place a mask on the patient to limit droplet dissemination; use insecticides, flea barriers, and rodent control measures so that the insect vectors don't bite the patient and spread the plague beyond your house. One paper advocates a Mosquito net around the patient. This probably should be done during summers, and insect season.
- The patient may want the bubo, if one exists, to be drained. Do *not* do it, because if not handled properly it can get into the skin of the one who is doing the drainage.
- Infected individuals in your home should have their own space with access restricted to caretakers. Isolation can be discontinued after 48 hours of appropriate antibiotic therapy.
- Immediate treatment is mandatory. Half of untreated patients with bubonic plague will die, as will virtually all of those with pneumonic plague. These numbers can be reduced to less than 5% and 20–40%, respectively, if antibiotic therapy starts within 18–24 hours of symptom onset.
- *Y. pestis* is fragile and can live for only an hour after aerosol release. Decontamination following aerosol release of the plague is unnecessary. Keep in mind, however, that some reports say the plague can live for 30 days in water, up to two years in moist ground, and up to a year in near-frozen ground. Survival varies with the environmental conditions, and you should not take the sterility of your environment for granted.

- Report suspected cases or suspected intentional release of the plague to your local health department. The local health department is responsible for notifying the state health department, the FBI, and local law enforcement. The state health department will notify the CDC.

3

Tularemia

Delivery: Inhalation or ingestion of aerosols or contact with a tick or other tularemia-infected arthropod or animal.

Symptoms: Starts as a sudden, flulike illness, including fever, malaise, and chills. Especially common are lower back pain and muscle ache, and headache. Half of those infected develop pulmonary symptoms, including cough (generally nonproductive) and chest pain. Can progress to multiorgan failure and death.

Timeline: Symptoms develop from 1 to 14 days following exposure, but usually between 3 and 5 days.

Can be mistaken for: Bubonic plague, anthrax, Q fever, and community-acquired pneumonia.

Treatment: The medication of choice is streptomycin, delivered through intramuscular (IM) route, or gentamicin, via IM or IV. Oral alternatives include doxycycline, chloramphenicol, and ciprofloxacin. Avoid penicillins and cephalosporins because they are not effective.

Tularemia in Nature

Often referred to as rabbit or deer fly fever, tularemia is a zoonosis, which means humans are infected by animals and not each other. Natural reservoirs, found throughout much of North America, include small mammals such as voles, mice, water rats, squirrels, rabbits, and hares. Naturally acquired human infection occurs through a variety of means, including tick bite, handling of infectious animal tissues or fluids; direct contact with or ingestion of contaminated water, food, or soil; and inhalation of infective aerosols. *F. tularensis* is so infective that inhalation of as few as ten organisms can cause disease, as can examining an open plate of culture.

The disease was discovered in 1911 in Tulare, California, as the bacterial cause of a plaguelike illness in ground squirrels. Human forms of the disease were identified in 1914, and it was shown to be transmitted by deerflies as well as infected blood. Notable for multiple sporadic outbreaks but no large epidemics, the disease is endemic in rural areas in moderate climates, particularly in the midwestern United States. The Soviets suggested naming the genus *Francisella* after Edward Francis, the researcher who helped to clarify our understanding of the disease, and so *Francisella tularensis* became its official name.

Tularemia as a Weapon of Biological Terror

Tularemia is an ideal means of biological terror because it can be contracted through simple breathing, and can remain viable in the environment for weeks and frozen for years. Aerosol dissemination of the species *Francisella tularensis* in a populated area would probably result, some 3 to 5 days later, in the abrupt appearance of thousands of patients with flu. Without antibiotic treatment, the clinical course for 30 to 60% of these victims could progress to respiratory failure, shock, and death. With treatment, the mortality rate would fall to 2%. In 1970, the World Health Organization (WHO) reported that 50 kilograms of virulent *F. tularensis*, dispersed as aerosol over a metropolitan area with a population of 5 million, would kill 19,000 and incapacitate 250,000 others. Clearly, swift recognition and immediate antibiotic treatment would save many thousands of lives.

F. tularensis, the bacterial organism that causes tularemia, is one of the most infectious pathogens known, requiring inoculation or inhalation of as few as ten organisms to cause disease. According to the Johns Hopkins Working Group on Civilian Biodefense, it is considered to be a dangerous potential biological weapon because of its extreme infectivity, ease of dissemination, and substantial capacity to cause illness and death.

During World War II, a host of nations, including Japan and the United States, studied *F. tularensis* and its utility as a biological weapon. Most people don't know, however, that tularemia may have been decisive in winning the war for the Soviets, much as the atom bomb was decisive in the victory of the United States. History texts refer, often dramatically, to the battle of Stalingrad, where more than a million Soviet soldiers died fending off German invaders from what could have been their nation's last stand. The turning point of that struggle came late in the summer of 1942, when German panzer troops fell inexplicably ill, enabling the Soviets to push them back. Sick in epidemic number, the Germans had become temporarily incapacitated by tularemia, halting their ability to fight. That temporary hiatus was enough for Russian soldiers to force the Germans into retreat—even though the Russians thereafter came down with tularemia themselves.

Decades later, Soviet military scientist Ken Alibek, a trained epidemiologist, was intrigued by the odd epidemic, in which only one Army took ill at first. Investigating, he learned that the Soviets had indeed developed a tularemia weapon in a secret bacteriological weapons facility in the city of Kirov in 1941, the year before the Stalingrad siege. Reporting in his book, *Biohazard,* Alibeck says he has "no doubt that the weapon had been used."

Tularemia was one of several biological weapons stockpiled by the U.S. military in the late 1960s, then allegedly destroyed by 1973. The Soviet Union continued weapons production of antibiotic- and vaccine-resistant strains into the early 1990s.

In fact, Alibek says it was *his* group that created and tested what is likely the world's first vaccine-resistant tularemia weapon in 1991. In tests conducted two years in a row on Rebirth Island, a "tear-shaped speck" between Uzbekistan and Kazakhstan, in the Aral Sea, Alibek's team vaccinated monkeys for tularemia and then injected them with the disease. In what the Soviets called a great success, all the monkeys died.

Unless his vaccine-resistant tularemia is eventually used, Alibek's testimony may be the best evidence of this work we will ever have. At Rebirth Island, "everything connected to the tularemia test, from research notes to blood samples to the monkeys' corpses had to be incinerated," he writes in his book. "The testing area was swept clean of all signs of human and animal occupation and then disinfected to eliminate all 'footprints' of biological activity."

Signs and Symptoms

Over the past decade, there have been fewer than 200 cases of tularemia in the United States. There are six types of tularemia, named for their symptoms and the route of exposure:

Ulceroglandular Tularemia   Characterized by skin ulcer and swollen glands. Occurs via contact with an infected animal (particularly rabbits) or by arthropod (particularly tick) bite. This is the most common form of the disease in nature, accounting for between 50 and 85% of cases. Less than 5% of those afflicted die, even without treatment.

Glandular Tularemia   About 10% of the cases seen in nature fall into this category, presenting with gland involvement but not skin ulcers. As with the ulceroglandular form of the disease, mortality without treatment is less than 5%.

Oculoglandular Tularemia   Characterized by conjunctivitis and local swelling following inoculation into the eye. Theoretically possible from aerosol or from direct contact with infected material. Less than 5% of cases result in death without treatment.

Oropharyngeal Tularemia   Pharyngitis (also known as tonsillitis, marked by extreme sore throat) and cervical swelling following ingestion of inadequately cooked meat from an infected animal.

Typhoidal Tularemia   Presents as severe systemic disease without skin ulcers, swelling of glands, or pneumonia. Any route of infection is possible. This category accounts for between 5 and 15% of tularemia cases. This form of the disease could be an outcome of bioterrorism. Mortality without treatment can reach 30–60%.

Pneumonic Tularemia   In nature, this form accounts for just 5% of tularemia cases, but it is the most likely presentation in any biological attack. Although up to half of all tularemia cases present with lung involvement from spread of systemic infection through the bloodstream, this term generally refers to lung infection resulting from direct inhalation of aerosolized bacteria. When untreated, 30–60% of those infected will die.

The major target organs for tularemia are the lymph nodes, the lungs, the spleen, the liver, and the kidneys. In the case of a bioterrorist aerosol attack, typhoidal and pneumonic tularemia are the varieties most likely to emerge. Both are notable for fever, headache, malaise, chest discomfort, and cough. In both forms of tularemia, a chest x-ray may show abnormalities in 50% of the affected.

How the Disease Is Diagnosed by Medical Professionals

According to authoritative literature, medical professionals should diagnose tularemia clinically—a relatively difficult feat considering how few have ever seen a case in their practice. Nonetheless, experts recommend clinical diagnosis based on symptoms, especially in the presence of a known tularemia outbreak, because the organism is not only difficult but also dangerous to culture, often causing disease in the lab workers themselves. Physicians who opt for testing, therefore, often rely on serology tests—blood tests that measure antibodies to invading infections. Measurable antibody levels are said to appear within a week of infection, but levels high enough for specific diagnosis require 2 weeks—a long time in a rapidly moving illness whose endpoint can be death. What's more, even a positive test is questionable, since antibodies to *F. tularensis* may cross-react with other infections, including *Brucella*, *Proteus,* and *Yersinia* organisms, and because detectable antibody levels may persist for many years after a bout of tularemia.

While these tests may be useful guideposts for doctors, the clinical picture is the most important where tularemia is concerned. The bottom line is this: there are currently no widely available rapid confirmatory diagnostic tests for tularemia. A presumptive diagnosis can be made quickly based on presenting symptoms if there is a high index of suspicion. Blood, saliva, biopsy specimens, and eye fluids may all be used to aid in diagnosis.

Care and Treatment

Antibiotic therapy is the appropriate treatment for tularemia. According to the Working Group on Civilian Biodefense, made up of 25 representatives from academic medical centers, civilian and military governmental agencies, and other public health and emergency management institutions and agencies, the first choices for treatment in the event of attack are intravenous (IV) and intramuscular (IM) antibiotics of the sort dispersed from the hospital. The Working Group published their recommendations in the *Journal of the American Medical Association* in June 2001 based on their review of peer-reviewed literature, as summarized below:

Adults, Preferred Choices

- Streptomycin, 1 gram IM every 12 hours for 10 days.
- Gentamicin, 5 mg/kg IV or IM once a day every day for 10 days.
- Ciprofloxacin, 400 mg IV twice daily for 10 days.

Adults, Aternative Treatments

- Doxycycline, 100 mg IV twice daily for 14–21 days.
- Chloramphenicol, 15 mg/kg IV four times daily for 14–21 days.
- Ciprofloxacin, 15 mg/kg IV twice daily for 10 days.

Children, Preferred Choices

- Streptomycin, 15 mg/kg IM every 12 hours for 10 days. Up to two grams per day.
- Gentamicin, 2.5 mg/kg IV or IM three times a day every day for 10 days.

Children, Alternative Choices

- Doxycycline, 100 mg IV twice daily for 14–21 days if weight is greater than 100 pounds; 2.2 mg/kg IV twice daily for 14–21 days if weight is less than 100 pounds.
- Chloramphenicol, 15 mg/kg IV four times daily for 14–21 days.
- Ciprofloxacin, 15 mg/kg IV four times daily for 10 days.

Pregnant Women, Preferred Choices

- Gentamicin, 5 mg/kg IV or IM once a day every day for 10 days. The Working Group notes that gentamicin poses a particularly low risk to the fetus.
- Streptomycin, 1 g IM every 12 hours for 10 days.

Pregnant Women, Alternative Choices

- Doxycycline, 100 mg IV twice daily for 14–21 days.
- Ciprofloxacin, 400 mg IV twice daily for 10 days.

Further note: While streptomycin has historically been the drug of choice for tularemia, it may not be available owing to small production runs (you can try to locate some by contacting the Roerig Streptomycin Program at Pfizer Pharmaceuticals in New York at 800-254-4445). But beyond that, streptomycin may not be the best choice. Indeed, a fully virulent streptomycin-resistant strain of *F. tularensis* was developed by the Soviet Union during the 1950s and it is presumed that other countries have obtained it. The strain was sensitive to gentamicin, however. And gentamicin offers the advantage of providing broader coverage that extends to other bacteria, and may be useful when the diagnosis of tularemia is in doubt. The Working Group therefore recommends that gentamicin and other alternatives be considered before streptomycin.

Of course, in the event of a bioterrorist attack, the public health care system may be too overwhelmed or undersupplied to handle your case with IV or IM treatment for any antibiotic at all. In that case, oral antibiotics will have to do—as long as you avoid penicillin and cephalosporins, which are known to be ineffective against tularemia. The Working Group recommends the following:

Adults

- Ciprofloxacin, 500 mg every 12 hours for 2 weeks.
- Doxycycline, 100 mg every 12 hours for 2 weeks.

Children

- Ciprofloxacin, 15 mg/kg every 12 hours for 2 weeks.

- Doxycyclinc, 100 mg every 12 hours for 2 weeks if more than 100 pounds. If less than 100 pounds, 2.2 mg/kg twice daily.

Pregnant Women

- Ciprofloxacin, 500 mg every 12 hours for 2 weeks. This is the best alternative for pregnant women if IV or IM gentamicin are unavailable.
- Doxycycline, 100 mg every 12 hours for 2 weeks.

For all age groups, Cipro has a lower relapse rate than doxycyline.

The mere presence of tularemia in your community does not mean you have been exposed or infected, or that you need treatment, even if you have some symptoms of the disease. "Other, more common diseases will still be present," Dr. Paul Rega of the Center for Bioterrorism Preparedness notes, "so evaluation at a health care center is essential." Treatment guidelines in force at the time will differentiate between those who are at risk for tularemia and those who clearly have something as simple as the flu.

That said, if it's been determined you were exposed within a few days of a known attack, prophylatic treatment is called for. Experts recommend a two-week course of oral antibodies, at the same dosage recommended for infection. If you start the treatment within 24 hours of exposure, you may escape symptoms of disease.

"In the unlikely event that authorities quickly become aware that an *F. tularensis* biological weapon has been used and are able to identify and reach exposed persons during the early incubation period," the Working Group recommends that "exposed persons be prophylactically treated with 14 days of oral doxycycline or ciprofloxacin. In a circumstance in which the weapon attack has been covert and the event is discovered only after persons start to become ill, then anyone potentially exposed should be instructed to begin a fever watch. Persons who develop an otherwise unexplained fever or flulike illness within 14 days of presumed exposure should begin treatment for the disease."

If you may have been exposed but are not given prophylaxis, Dr. Rega recommends that you monitor your fever a couple of times a day and return to the doctor if your temperature reaches 100 degrees Fahrenheit. If the doctor insists upon waiting for laboratory confirmation, even though you are symptomatic and may have been exposed, demand that he or she call the local or state health department or CDC for their specific protocols and directives before releasing you from their care. If you do not get the service or answers you feel comfortable with from your personal physician, clinic, or emergency department, Dr. Rega emphasizes, then you must call a higher authority for input.

Note: Prophylactic treatment is not recommended following potential natural exposure from ticks, rabbits, or other animals, but it is recommended in the event of a bioterrorism attack.

As to vaccine protection, there is none at the current time for civilian populations. An experimental vaccine, however, has been given to more than 5,000 people; significant adverse reactions have not occurred. But experts warn that even this vaccine might not guard against infection if an individual is overwhelmed by extremely high doses of the tularemia bacterium.

Since there is no known human-to-human transmission, neither isolation nor quarantine is required, and you can care for your loved ones without fear of infection yourself. Use disinfectants for soiled clothing, bedding, equipment, and so on. Heat and disinfectants easily inactivate the organism.

What You Need to Know to Survive an Attack of Tularemia

- Intentional aerosol release of tularemia should be suspected if cases occur in nonendemic areas when no discernible risk factors for exposure are identified.
- It is inappropriate to base a tularemia diagnosis on a laboratory test of any kind. Especially in the setting of an outbreak or a bioterrorism event, physicians must base diagnosis on symptoms and the likelihood or possibility of exposure. If your physician insists upon laboratory confirmation under these conditions, seek other medical help immediately.
- Early symptoms usually appear in 2–5 days and up to 21 days after exposure, and present as a sudden flu, complete with fever, chills, headache, cough, elevated white blood cell count, and generalized body aches.

- Tularemia cannot be transmitted from person to person, so you need not fear exposure by caring for a loved one with the disease.
- Tularemia can survive for weeks in water, soil, and animal carcasses and is resistant to freezing temperatures, but is easily eradicated on surfaces by heat (55°C or 131°F for 10 minutes) or standard disinfectants.
- Treatment should be initiated as soon as a diagnosis of tularemia is suspected and should not be delayed for confirmatory testing. Cure rates are high if antibiotics are started prior to development of severe illness.
- If you are sick or fear you have been exposed, begin antibiotic therapy with the recommended medications at the recommended dose. In a true emergency, it is unlikely you will be able to obtain first-line medications such as streptomycin and gentamicin, but remember that you may also use such standbys as doxycycline and Cipro.
- If symptoms persist after treatment, ask your physician to culture your blood for the organism. Tularemia has been cultured from blood following antibiotic treatment, indicating the organism can persist. In this case, you may require another round of treatment.
- If authorities quickly become aware that an *F. tularensis* biological weapon has been used and are able to identify you as one of the exposed during the early incubation period, you should be treated prophylactically with 14 days of oral doxycycline or ciprofloxacin.
- If a tularemia attack has been covert, and if the event is thus discovered only after persons start to become ill, anyone who has been potentially exposed should be instructed to begin a fever watch. Persons who develop an otherwise unexplained fever or flu-like illness within 14 days of presumed exposure should begin treatment for the disease.
- If you have been exposed but are not given prophylaxis, monitor your fever a couple of times a day and return to the doctor to request evaluation for treatment at once if your temperature reaches 100 degrees Fahrenheit.
- Should the doctor insist upon waiting for laboratory confirmation even though you are symptomatic and may have been exposed to tularemia in a bioterrorist attack, demand that he call the local or state health department or CDC for their specific protocols and directives before releasing you from his care.

- Report suspected cases or suspected intentional release of tularemia to your local health department. The local health department is responsible for notifying the state health department, the FBI, and local law enforcement. The state health department will notify the CDC.

4

Cholera

Delivery: Ingestion of contaminated food or water.

Symptoms: Initially presents with vomiting, distended stomach, and headache. But the hallmark symptom is voluminous diarrhea. Without treatment, fluid loss is so significant that death can result from dehydration.

Timeline: Symptoms develop anywhere from a few hours to 5 days after ingesting the organism.

Can be mistaken for: *E. coli,* and *Vibrio parahaemolyticus,* different bacteria with the same symptoms, requiring similar treatment. Other organisms that may be confused with cholera include rotavirus, staphylococcal enterotoxin B (SEB), a deadly bacterial toxin, and *Bacillus* cereus, a spore-forming bacterium associated with food poisoning.

Treatment: Rapid, aggressive oral rehydration and antibiotics, especially tetracycline.

Cholera in Nature

The author Gabriel Garcia Marquez called it right when he entitled his novel of romantic heartache *Love in the Time of Cholera*. In terms of meting out swift judgment, unbridled tragedy, and cruel twists of fate, the rod-shaped bacterial agent *Vibrio cholerae* is virtually unchallenged on earth. Producing severe, often lethal dehydration through release of a toxin, *V. cholarae* has historically devastated populations worldwide by infiltrating water supplies and the food chain.

Cholera pandemics were common in the 19th and early 20th century, including one that began in Indonesia in 1961 and spread rapidly until it ran out of steam in South America in 1991. Cholera outbreaks still occur worldwide due to reservoirs of infection in the environment. Some of the more prominent local habitats for *V. cholerae* include brackish estuaries along the Louisiana and Texas coast and the Gulf of Mexico. The route to natural infection is consumption of raw or undercooked fish.

Cholera as a Weapon of Biological Terror

Intentional use of cholera by terrorists would presumably involve contamination of food or water supplies. For those who prefer this route of delivery, cholera could be the bioweapon of choice.

It was appealing to the Japanese, for instance, when they conducted their biological weapons research in occupied Manchuria between 1932 and 1945. During this period, Japan launched biological attacks on at least 11 Chinese cities, deploying infectious agents by directly contaminating water and food supplies, among other routes. Although they used a host of biological weapons, in a single attack on Changteh in 1941, 10,000 Chinese citizens and 1,700 Japanese troops died, predominantly from cholera.

The Germans had a penchant for cholera, too. Although they were much more comfortable with chemical than biological weapons, they still put effort into developing weaponized cholera, even using it to attack Italy in 1915, according to charges made. The Japanese, meanwhile, claimed they had recovered bottles of weaponized cholera from Russian spies.

Signs and Symptoms

Once an individual has been exposed to cholera, the incubation period to onset of symptoms is between 1 and 5 days. The degree of sickness varies with the patient. Persons infected with *V. cholerae* may be asymptomatic, have mild diarrhea, or full-blown disease characterized by sudden onset of vomiting and abdominal cramping and distension followed by profuse watery diarrhea. Clearly, given these symptoms, one can expect rapid loss of body fluids and frequent collapse. After several watery bowel movements the stools take on a "rice-water" appearance. Low blood pressure may set in within an hour of the first symptoms.

At its most extreme, the stool volume generated by cholera is greater than that associated with any other gastrointestinal disease, and victims can lose up to 5 or 10 liters of fluid a day. The patient can become dehydrated and go into shock within hours.

Even the sickest patients usually do not have a fever.

How the Disease Is Diagnosed by Medical Professionals

In the hospital, the cholera patient will receive appropriate diagnostic tests. These include dark-field microscopy of cholera stools, which reveal large numbers of vibrios (short, curved rods) with a characteristic motility that gives the appearance of shooting stars. Cultures are often made directly from stool or from a rectal swab. While specimens are sent out for laboratory confirmation, physicians can perform other, supportive tests. For instance, stool samples seldom will have red or white cells on microscopic examination. But given the swift blows dealt by this disease, treatment cannot wait for confirmation from a lab.

Care and Treatment

Cholera leads to dehydration and electrolyte loss. These two conditions account for virtually all signs and symptoms, ultimately causing hypoglycemia (shortage of glucose in the blood), hypokalemia (potassium deficiency), cardiac arrest, shock, and death. Progression from the first symptoms to shock and then death can be swift, with shock appearing 4–12 hours after onset and death following from 18 hours to several days later. Those in the hospital will receive immediate intravenous treatment with antibiotics and lactated Ringer's (LR) solution for persistent vomiting or high rates of stool loss. Oral rehydration solution (ORS) is added to the treatment in the hospital setting as well.

If you contract cholera and find yourself under care at the hospital, consider yourself blessed. The fact of the matter is, however, that a terrorist event, depending upon its magnitude, could leave you to your own resources for a couple of days or more.

Should that happen, you'd do well to have some oral rehydration solutions of your own on hand. Your best bet will be the World Health Organization solution, available from Jianas Brothers Packaging in Kansas City, which contains glucose and a specific mix of salts. Other recommended brands include Naturalyte, Rehydralyte, Infolyte, and Pedialyte.

Mild and moderately dehydrated patients should be instructed to drink ORS until they are no longer thirsty. Daily oral replacement volume should include ongoing losses plus 1 liter; adults may need over 5 liters of fluid a day. Children are to receive 5–10 cubic centimeters of solution by syringe every 5–10 minutes. The patient's rehydration status should be reassessed every 1–2 hours.

If you are caring for a cholera patient at home, you can assess rehydration status through the following guide:

- Still fairly hydrated: mentally awake and alert; eyes bright and clear; tears present and mouth moist, even if somewhat thirsty; skin taut; urine output same as usual (color: light); pulse present and full, even if a little fast; breathing, same as usual.
- Moderately dehydrated: restless and irritable; dull affect, though still somewhat responsive; eyes sunken, with minimal tearing. May complain of severe thirst; urine output decreased and dark (concentrated); skin, loose; pulse faster, with diminished strength; breathing faster.
- Severely dehydrated: lethargic and unresponsive; eyes very sunken, with no tears; no moisture in mouth; skin very loose and dry; no urine output; pulse not palpable; breathing may go from very fast to an ominous slowdown as death approaches.

It may be difficult to obtain oral rehydrating solution from the World Health Organization in the midst of a catastrophic cholera attack. If you are unable to obtain this formulation, you should try to buy other recommended brands, which will be more useful than plain water.

Remember that, as caretaker, it is your job to help hydrate the cholera patient, but you should not do so by attempting to stop the diarrhea. The World Health Organization recommends that you avoid any anti-diarrheal agents you might have in your medicine cabinet. For the cholera patient, correct rehydration could determine ultimate survival, so your best bet is attempting it under the guidance of a health care professional, if one is available.

If you or a loved one develops symptoms of cholera, or if you hear of a cholera attack in your area and believe you have been exposed, you should begin treatment with antibiotics, as follows:

Adults

- 500 mg tetracycline every 6 hours for 3 days.
- 300 mg doxycycline once a day for 3 days.
- 100 mg doxycycline twice a day for 3 days (this protocol is shown to shorten the duration of diarrhea and reduce fluid losses).

Other antibiotics can be considered as well if the above protocols do not work due to presumed, widespread tetracycline resistance. These include:

- 1000 mg of ciprofloxacin as a one-time dose.
- 500 mg of ciprofloxacin every 12 hours for 3 days.
- 500 mg of erythromycin every 6 hours for 3 days.
- 400 mg of norfloxacin every 12 hours for 3 days.
- 250 mg of ampicillin every 6 hours for 5 days.

Children

- 50 mg/kg of tetracycline divided into 4 doses for 3 days. Not to exceed 2 grams a day.
- 40 mg/kg erythromycin divided into 4 doses for 3 days.
- 8 mg trimethoprim and 40 mg/kg sulfamethoxazole divided into 2 doses a day for 3 days.
- 5 mg/kg furazolidone divided into 4 doses for 3 days.

A cholera vaccine is available but not recommended, because it protects only approximately half of those vaccinated, and because it provides only short-term immunity. Moreover, since the vaccine takes weeks to become effective, it would be useless during a cholera epidemic.

What You Need to Know to Survive an Attack of Cholera

- Symptoms of cholera are the result of fluid loss. Therefore, make sure patients are rehydrated with appropriate fluids as soon as possible.
- Make sure that infants are never hydrated with plain water, since it can push them to seizure under conditions of dehydration. Instead, you must rehydrate babies with Pedialyte.
- Untreated cholera kills 50% of its victims, but less than 1% of those treated with antibiotics and rehydration fluids succumb to the disease.
- Tetracycline is the drug of choice for treating cholera in both children and adults.
- Tetracycline-resistant strains of cholera are prevalent. Be aware that weaponized cholera may be resistant to tetracycline. If you come in contact with such a strain, Cipro is the drug of choice.
- If there has been an outbreak of cholera, make sure to boil all water and adequately cook all food to kill the organism.
- Proper hygiene is essential for anyone caring for a patient suffering from cholera. This is because transmission occurs through the fecal-oral route and could potentially be spread from the contaminated stool or vomitus of infected cases. Nonetheless, person-to-person transmission is unlikely when precautions are taken to avoid contact.
- Proper hand washing after using the rest room and before preparing or eating food is critical to decrease chance of transmission.
- If contaminated water is the source, all beverages and foods associated with the water source are considered contaminated and should be avoided, including ice, sauces, or pastas and grains that required water for preparation and foods rinsed with the contaminated water.
- *Vibrio cholerae* is readily killed by dry heat at 242°F, by steam, through boiling, or by short exposure to ordinary disinfectants and chlorination of water.

- Any person who shared food or drink with a cholera patient should be under surveillance for 5 days, and objects contaminated with feces or vomit should be disinfected prior to reuse.
- Report suspected cases or suspected intentional release of cholera to your local health department. The local health department is responsible for notifying the state health department, the FBI, and local law enforcement. The state health department will notify the CDC.

5

Q Fever

Delivery: Inhalation of aerosol or ingestion of contaminated food or water.

Symptoms: Initially presents as the flu, with headache, chills, lethargy, and profuse sweating. Pneumonia occurs in half the victims, and may present with or without cough and respiratory symptoms. Look also for nausea and vomiting. Goes on to manifest a host of neurological symptoms, including but not limited to double vision, encephalitis (a swelling of the brain), and hallucinations.

Timeline: Symptoms develop anywhere from 10 to 40 days after exposure, but usually within 2 weeks. Illness usually lasts from 2 days to 2 weeks, but can last for months in up to 30% of victims.

Can be mistaken for: Pneumonia, brucellosis, tularemia, plague, babesiosis. Also, a host of viral illnesses, including *Mycoplasma pneumoniae*, *Legionella pneumophila*, *Chlamydia psittaci*, and *Chlamydia pneumoniae*.

Treatment: The antibiotics tetracycline and doxycycline.

Q Fever in Nature

Q fever, also known as "query" fever, results in nature when the rickettsia *Coxiella burnetii* is transferred from farm animals to people. The farm animals themselves, including goats, sheep, and cows, are usually asymptomatic, but they can transfer the infection to other species, including dogs, cats, rodents, some birds, and humans. Naturally occurring human disease is rare, however, and found mostly in veterinarians, sheep or meat workers, and farmers; individuals from endemic areas with no animal contact have, from time to time, come down with Q fever as well.

Q fever is transmitted by inhalation of aerosolized particles from the tissues, fluids, or waste products of infected animals or from direct contact with contaminated materials. Since the microbes gravitate to the placenta, handling fetal material or tissue or any products of conception puts workers at especially high risk.

Q Fever as a Weapon of Biological Terror

Coxiella burnetii is resistant to heat and desiccation and highly infectious by the aerosol route. A single inhaled organism may produce clinical illness. For these reasons, Q fever could be a highly effective and incapacitating agent of biological war. Indeed, it has been estimated that 50 kilograms of dried, powdered *C. burnetii* would produce casualties at a rate equal to that of similar amounts of anthrax or tularemia organisms.

The potential of Q fever to wreak havoc has long been recognized by both the United States and the USSR. In 1954, when the Army's Chemical Corps received permission to use human volunteers in the evaluation of biological agents, aerosolized *C. Burnetii* was subjected to open-air tests of 30 people at Dugway Proving Ground, Utah. Munitions and stocks (except that required for vaccine research) were publicly destroyed by executive order of President Richard M. Nixon between May 1971 and May 1972. In August 1992, the *Washington Post* reported claims of a confidential report on the extent of the Russian biological weapons program by Anatoly Kuntsevich, a retired Russian general and a former director of Soviet research on chemical arms. Kuntsevich stated in the report that the military had illicitly developed aerial bombs and rocket warheads. These warheads were capable of carrying several biological warfare agents, he said, including anthrax, tularemia, and Q fever. He maintained that the biological weapons effort had been maintained through at least 1990 but had been scaled down during the 6 years of Mikhail Gorbachev's presidency. Whether the program was actually scaled down in 1990, and whether stockpiles remain, is currently unknown.

Signs and Symptoms

According to biowarfare experts, intentional release by a terrorist would probably involve aerosolization of the organism and case presentation would be similar to naturally occurring disease. While physicians in endemic areas might be adept at noting an increase in cases and identifying weaponized Q fever, diagnosis would be more difficult in urban locales.

The reason is that the symptoms can be general and diffuse. Disease begins with the sudden onset of fever, chills, headache, weakness, lethargy, anorexia, and profuse sweating. Pneumonia occurs in approximately half of the cases and may be present without accompanying respiratory symptoms such as cough, expectoration, or chest pain. If there has been a Q fever attack in your area, expect infection to incubate anywhere from 9 to 39 days before symptoms emerge, although the average period is 2 or 3 weeks.

While temporarily debilitating, the disease usually resolves without treatment, and only 1% of the untreated die. It presents extreme danger only to one significant group: pregnant women and their unborn children. Indeed, since the *Coxiella burnetii* bacteria gravitate to the placenta, exposure may lead to high rates of fetal infection and miscarriage.

About one-third of Q fever victims will develop acute hepatitis. This can present with fever and abnormal liver function tests with the absence of pulmonary signs and symptoms. Uncommon complications include chronic hepatitis, culture-negative endocarditis (inflammation of the heart), aseptic meningitis, encephalitis (inflammation of the brain), and osteomyelitis (inflammation of the bone marrow and adjacent bone). Most patients who develop endocarditis have preexisting valvular heart disease.

Most of those who go without treatment clear the infection on their own, but a small percentage go on to develop endocarditis and chronic infection. From 30 to 60% of these individuals will die without treatment. They can be cured but require more aggressive therapy with a combination of antibiotics.

While Q fever is merciful compared to other weaponized germs, it is still a weapon of choice. The reason is that what Q fever lacks in lethality it makes up in ease of delivery and in the sheer potential to wreak havoc for weeks. It is, in many ways, the ideal weaponized germ because it naturally withstands heat and drying. Just a single microbe can cause disease. Q fever may not kill the enemy, but it can be used to destabilize and panic a population since its early symptoms are similar to those of anthrax and might be confused for that deadly disease.

How Medical Experts Diagnose the Disease

Diagnosis is difficult because Q fever is often nonspecific in presentation—a fever of unknown origin and pneumonia, after all, can come from many infections, viral and bacterial alike. Laboratory confirmation of the diagnosis is possible only some 2–3 weeks after onset of symptoms, when antibodies have risen enough for detection. Polymerase chain reaction tests can be used to identify organisms through analysis of DNA in tissue or environmental samples. A Western Blot test can be used to identify chronic versions of the disease by detecting antibodies in the blood.

Care and Treatment

If you find you have contracted Q fever, you must be treated at once. If you learn there has been an outbreak of Q fever in your area, you must make sure you receive prophylactic treatment—but not immediately. Here, timing is everything, medical studies show. The optimum time to start prophylactic treatment for Q fever is 8–12 days after exposure. Prophylaxis provided immediately postexposure delays onset of symptoms but does not prevent infection.

Recommended treatment for this disease is:

Adults

- 500 mg of tetracycline every 6 hours for 15–21 days (7 days for mild illness).
- 100 mg of doxycycline morning and night for 15–21 days (7 days for mild illness).

Children Under 100 Pounds

- 40 mg/kg of tetracycline four times a day for 15–21 days (7 days for mild illness).
- 4–5 mg/kg doxycycline twice a day for 15–21 days (7 days for mild illness).

Pregnant Women

- Co-trimoxazole, 1 double strength tablet every 12 hours for 15–21 days. Avoid this treatment if patient is at term. Co-trimoxazole, also known as TMP/SMX, is a combination of two antibiotics— trimethoprim and sulfamethoxazole. It is sold under the brand names Bactrim and Septra.
- Ciprofloxacin, 500 mg every 12 hours for 15–21 days.

Prophylaxis

Use tetracycline or doxycycline as above, but start 8–12 days after exposure and continue for 5 days.

Finally, for those with endocarditis and chronic infection, combination antibiotic treatment must be continued for a period of at least 24 months, according to William R. Byrne, M.D., Chief, Genetics and Physiology Branch, Bacteriology Division, U.S. Army Medical Research Institute of Infectious Diseases, Fort Detrick, Maryland. Even with treatment, 24% of these patients die, and for a complete cure, valve replacement is often required. The following protocols have worked:

- 500 mg erythromycin four times a day with 600 mg rifampin once a day.
- 500 mg of tetracycline every 6 hours and 600 mg rifampin once a day.
- 100 mg of doxycycline morning and night and 600 mg rifampin once a day.

For those who cannot take doxycycline or tetracycline, Cipro is an appropriate alternative, according to the U.S. Army's *Medical Management of Biological Casualties Handbook,* produced at Fort Detrick.

If you have been exposed to a direct release of the Q fever, pay care-

ful attention to techniques for decontamination. Q fever is highly stable
and is resistant to heat and many disinfectants. Exposed individuals
should wash their skin with soap and water, and their clothing should be
handled carefully to avoid aerosolization and possible transmission during removal and laundry (this does not apply if the exposure is discovered retrospectively). Exposed individuals are those that were exposed
to the initial release; person-to-person transmission does not occur.

As to vaccination, none is available to the general public, although
an experimental vaccine is available and recommended for lab, abattoir,
or research employees working with sheep or *Coxiella burnetii*. A skin
sensitivity test should be provided before vaccine administration; the
vaccine should not be given to those with a positive skin test or those
with a history of Q fever disease.

What You Need to Know to Survive an Attack of Q fever

- If you have been victim of an overt attack of Q fever, immediately
  undress and shower with plenty of soap. If the Q fever agent,
  Coxiella burnetii, has been in contact with your skin for more than
  30 minutes, rinse with 70% ethyl alcohol. Use 0.5% household
  bleach for any gross or visible contamination.
- Contaminated clothing may be a source of infection. Since organisms are resistant to heat, and it takes just a single microbe to
  cause disease, it may be best to discard these garments.
- You may clean any contaminated areas of your home with 0.5%
  bleach.
- Before cleaning your home or workplace, or while tending to a
  loved one, make sure you are wearing gloves, face mask, and protective gown.
- Q fever presents extreme danger only to one significant group—
  pregnant women and their unborn children. This is because *C. burnetii* gravitates to the placenta, with exposure leading to high rates
  of fetal infection and miscarriage.
- If you are sick or fear you have been exposed, begin antibiotic therapy with the recommended medications at the recommended dose
  and time.

- For maximum impact, those without symptoms should start prophylactic therapy 8 days after exposure.
- Report suspected cases or suspected intentional release of Q fever to the health department, the FBI, and local law enforcement. The state health department will notify the CDC.

Brucellosis

Delivery: Ingestion, inhalation of aerosols, or sabotage of the food supply.

Symptoms: Many of those infected with brucellosis remain asymptomatic, and those who become ill tend to present with non-specific symptoms including fever, headache, body aches, chills, profuse sweating, depression, weight loss, generalized weakness, and lethargy. Gastrointestinal (GI) symptoms are the most common complaint, with 70% of patients presenting with anorexia, nausea, vomiting, abdominal pain, and diarrhea or constipation. Cough and chest pain from infected lungs is seen in about 20% of patients. This might be higher with aerosol attack.

Timeline: Symptoms develop from 5 to 60 days following exposure, though most commonly between 8 and 14 days.

Can be mistaken for: The flu or any number of other infectious diseases, including plague, tularemia, Q fever, and Lyme disease.

Treatment: The standard of care involves 6 weeks of combination therapy with doxycycline, streptomycin, and rifampin for adults or 4–6 weeks with doxycycline or tetracycline for children.

Brucellosis in Nature

Most people know Florence Nightingale as the founder of modern nursing. Less well known is the fact that after her return from the Crimean War in 1856 she suffered inexplicable illness, becoming an invalid and, in the eyes of many contemporaries, a hypochondriac and malingerer. To experts of the day, the notion that her ills were psychosomatic seemed reasonable. The symptoms were, after all, vague, including weakness, headache, nausea at the sight of food, breathlessness, heart palpitations, and pain. But was Florence Nightingale simply stricken by stress-induced neurosis, or was she actually ill?

It took more than a century for medical science to weigh in anew on this issue, but from the perspective of 2002, an opinion has emerged: history's most renowned nurse probably suffered from brucellosis, the bacterial infection also said to cause "Crimean fever," the debilitating disease encountered by the British army in Malta during the Crimean War. Defined at the time as a remitting and relapsing illness, Crimean fever was characterized by nervous irritability, including fever and delirium and prolonged gastrointestinal irritation. With both remission and relapse common, the course of the disease was irregular and often protracted, with months of convalescence required. Even after so-called recovery, moreover, symptoms could persist for years.

It was in 1887 that Crimean fever was traced to the bacterium *Brucella melitensis*, identified by David Bruce. Other experts later identified goat milk as a reservoir of the infection, stating it could be transmitted through milk and milk products.

Today, according to the *British Medical Journal*, we know that the disease is caused not just by *B. melitensis*, but also by several other bacteria of the genus *Brucella,* with the specific course of disease dependent upon which species is involved. Remarkably persistent, *Brucella* bacteria can live in intracellular spaces hidden from the protective power of the immune system, explaining why symptoms may reemerge or simply continue for years.

Brucellosis as a Weapon of Biological Terror

Brucellosis is often considered low on the totem pole as a weapon of biological war. It has a long and variable incubation period, ranging from 5 to 60 days, making it unreliable and hard to predict. Many of those infected in natural epidemics remain asymptomatic, and the disease is rarely lethal; only 5% of the infected die. The disease is treatable with antibiotics.

Yet depending upon the strategy of the enemy, brucellosis could be a weapon of choice. One straightforward advantage is that it is highly infectious. It is estimated that inhalation of only 10 to 100 bacteria is sufficient to cause disease in humans. What's more, larger aerosol doses may shorten the incubation period and increase the clinical attack rate. And the disease is relatively prolonged, incapacitating, and disabling. While the targets may live, extreme physical illness and mental confusion may prevent them from mounting much of a counterattack while outside forces take control.

These traits were noted as long ago as 1942, when the United States began its effort to turn brucellosis into a weapon of war. The agent was manipulated to maintain long-term viability, placed into bombs, and tested in field trials with animals in 1944 and 1945. *Brucella* was also the first weaponized germ developed by the United States in its biological weapons program at Pine Bluff Arsenal in 1954. The weaponized *Brucella,* along with the remainder of America's biological arsenal, was destroyed in 1969, when the program was disbanded. But its potential for easy dispersal and its nonlethal, but devastating, effects place it on anyone's list of usual suspects as an agent of biological war.

Signs and Symptoms

Many people consider brucellosis primarily a veterinary disease, and in the Western Hemisphere, it largely is. Usually manifesting in animals, especially sheep, goats, and cattle, as an infection of the reproductive tract, it can cause spontaneous abortion or sterility. On the other hand, it's considered uncommon in humans and thus may be missed or easily misdiagnosed.

At first presenting as a flulike illness complete with fever, as in the Crimean War, it can later generate a host of specific, chronic symptoms, including arthritis and neurological effects, referred to as neurobrucellosis. In this version, brucellosis can spawn a wide spectrum of central and autonomic nervous system ills: tingling and numbness, motor disturbances, up to and including paralysis, and cognitive dysfunction, including memory loss and severe brain fog. Other chronic complications can include osteomyelitis (inflammation of the bone), epidydimitis (pelvic muscle strain), orchitis (inflammation of testicles), and endocarditis (infection of the endocardial surface of the heart).

Much like Florence Nightingale, those with chronic brucellosis can also suffer a series of vague symptoms, so generalized they are often difficult to differentiate from psychosomatic disease. These include insomnia, anorexia, nausea at the sight of food, anemia, nervousness, depression, delusions, palpitations, indigestion, headache, and nervous tremors. The longer the disease is active, according to the *British Medical Journal*, the more deeply entrenched these symptoms become.

A relapsing illness, chronic brucellosis can come and go over the course of time.

How the Disease Is Diagnosed by Medical Professionals

Because brucellosis is considered so rare in humans, doctors often need a high level of suspicion to make the connection. Human brucellosis is considered uncommon in the United States, with an annual incidence of 0.5 cases per 100,000 population. Most cases are associated with the ingestion of unpasteurized dairy products, or with abattoir and veterinary work. The disease is, however, highly endemic in Southwest Asia (annual incidence as high as 128 cases per 100,000 in some areas of Kuwait), thus representing a hazard to military personnel stationed in that theater.

To confirm their suspicion, doctors will send blood or bone marrow samples to a specialized lab that can culture *Brucella* organisms. Labs may also test the blood for antibodies against the infection. According to the CDC, since antibody levels may increase over time, two separate blood samples should be collected 2 weeks apart.

It should be noted that the tests can be inaccurate, yielding both false negatives and false positives. Indeed, laboratories culturing blood and bone marrow during the acute phase of the illness report finding microbes in anywhere from 15 to 70% of those who turn out to actually have the disease. Because of this, doctors have turned to the polymerase chain reaction test, which amplifies DNA, to get a more accurate reading of whether brucellosis is present.

Care and Treatment

Brucellosis requires about 6 weeks of treatment, usually with combination antibiotic therapy, and may frequently relapse after treatment. Without treatment, it may become a lifelong chronic disease. Most of the time, oral antibiotic therapy is the treatment of choice, though surgery may sometimes be required in uncommon cases of intense localized disease, especially the heart problem, endocarditis which results in the need for valve replacement.

The United States Army recommends the following:

- A combination of 200 mg of doxycycline a day by mouth and 600–900 mg of rifampin a day by mouth. Both should be divided into morning and evening doses, and should be taken for 6 weeks.
- As an alternative treatment, 200 mg of doxycycline a day by mouth for 6 weeks in combination 1 gram of streptomycin a day administered through intramuscular injection for 2 weeks.

According to the Center for the Study of Bioterrorism and Emerging Infections, St. Louis University School of Public Health, pregnant women should substitute doxycycline with TMP/SMX (the drug description for the two-antibiotic compound, trimethoprim/sulfamethoxazole, known also as co-trimoxazele and marketed under the names Bactrim and Septra).

For children, the St. Louis Center recommends the following:

- 2–4 mg/kg a day of liquid doxycycline, divided into two doses and taken by mouth for 4–6 weeks.
- 30–40 mg/kg of tetracycline taken by mouth for 4–6 weeks, age 8 and older.
- TMP/SMX in the following combination: trimethoprim 10mg/kg per day and sulfamethoxazole 50mg/kg per day, both by mouth, 4–6 weeks, age 8 and older.

Also studied and shown effective are regimens involving doxycycline plus gentamicin, TMP/SMX plus gentamicin, and ofloxacin plus rifampin. Long-term triple-drug therapy with rifampin, a tetracycline, and an aminoglycoside is recommended by some experts for patients with meningoencephalitis or endocarditis.

If you have been exposed to brucellosis in a natural setting, through contact with animals or milk, experts recommend that you do nothing. But if you have been exposed to weaponized or laboratory versions of the microbe, antibiotic treatment is a must. Here, the U.S. Army recommends a 3–6-week course of therapy with one of the regimens aforementioned.

What You Need to Know to Survive an Attack of Brucellosis

- You may show symptoms anywhere from 5 to 60 days after exposure.
- Symptoms may be vague in nature, starting with fever and flu, including headache, body aches, joint pain, and chills. Later symptoms may include depression, generalized weakness, and lethargy. Some 70% of patients have gastrointestinal symptoms, including nausea, abdominal pain, diarrhea, or constipation. Central nervous system disorders may include meningitis, encephalitis, and neuropathies, including numbness or tingling. In addition, an unknown neurotoxic process appears to cause severe behavioral changes in some patients.
- If you are tending an exposed loved one, rest assured that person-to-person transmission has not been reported through routine care. However, brucellosis can be transmitted through transfusion.
- *Brucella* may survive for 6 weeks in dust and up to 10 weeks in soil or water, but is easily killed by common disinfectants and heat.
- If you are sick or fear you have been exposed, begin antibiotic therapy with the recommended medications at the recommended dose and time.
- Report suspected cases or suspected intentional release of brucellosis to the health department, the FBI, and local law enforcement. The state health department will notify the CDC.

7
Glanders and Melioidosis

Delivery: Inhalation of aerosol.

Symptoms: High fever and multiorgan abscesses, predominantly in the lungs, liver, and spleen. Pulmonary symptoms, including bronchitis and pneumonia.

Timeline: Symptoms develop anywhere from 10 to 14 days after exposure.

Can be mistaken for: Tuberculosis, syphilis, and plague.

Treatment: Therapy will vary with the type and severity of the clinical presentation. Patients with localized disease may be managed with oral antibiotics for a duration of 60–150 days. More severe illness may require intravenous or intramuscular therapy and more prolonged treatment. Without treatment, 100% of the infected die within a month.

Glanders and Melioidosis in Nature

In nature, glanders is a horse disease caused by the bacillus bacteria, *Burkholderia mallei*. Rarely, humans in Asia, the Middle East, and South America contract the disease after handling infected horses, donkeys, or mules. Other than laboratory employees who fell ill with glanders at work, there have been no naturally acquired cases of the disease in the United States in over 61 years.

Much of what is true about glanders also holds for melioidosis, caused by *Burkholderia pseudomallei,* also a bacillus bacteria with a "safety-pin" appearance on microscopic examination. Both pathogens affect domestic and wild animals, which, like humans, acquire the diseases from inhalation or contaminated injuries. Members of the same genus, both cause disease with relatively similar symptoms and outcomes. Both are diagnosed and treated in similar fashion as well.

But while *B. mallei* inhabits a mammalian reservoir and rarely infects humans in the environment, *B. pseudomallei* is widely distributed in many tropical and subtropical regions and is, in fact, endemic in Southeast Asia and northern Australia. Melioidosis regularly infects humans in several distinct forms, ranging from a subclinical illness to an overwhelming infection, with a 90% mortality rate and death within 24 to 48 hours after onset. And while glanders is rarely seen in human populations at all, melioidosis not only is common but also can reactivate years after primary infection and result in chronic and life-threatening disease.

One of the principal reasons for their different profiles could well be their divergent habitats. While the organism causing glanders exists in nature only in infected animal hosts, the microbe causing melioidosis lives primarily in soil and dirt.

Glanders and Melioidosis as Weapons of Bioterrorism

Even though most of us have never even heard of glanders, it remains one of the top candidates for bioterrorism today. Its wrath in this regard was first felt during World War I, when it is believed to have been used to infect horses and mules carrying supplies, and during World War II, when it was allegedly directed not just at horses but also at civilians and prisoners of war.

Given its near-100% lethality without treatment 3–4 weeks after symptoms start, and its ability to incapacitate prior to death, it is a bioweapon of choice.

One use during the early part of the 20th century was to infect the animals used for war. During World War I, glanders was spread by the Central Powers to infect large numbers of Russian horses and mules on the Eastern Front. This impeded troop and supply convoys as well as artillery movement, at that time dependent on horses and mules. Human cases in Russia increased with the infections after the Japanese deliberately infected horses, civilians, and prisoners of war with *B. mallei* at the Pinfang (China) Institute during World War II.

The United States studied this agent as a possible biowarfare weapon in 1943–44 but did not weaponize it. The former Soviet Union is believed to have been interested in *B. mallei* as a potential biowarfare agent after World War II.

Like glanders, melioidosis must be delivered in aerosol form for maximum impact. It has been studied by the Americans and Soviets for its potential to wage biological war. Its ability to live in water, soil, and dust, however, gives it a hypothetical advantage over its cousin, which cannot survive in the environment after initial release. These attributes have been noted by both the Americans and the Soviets, who have studied this organism for their arsenals of biological war. For this disease, like glanders, mortality is high even with antibiotic treatment. An experiment with hamsters showed that a single one of these organisms, delivered by aerosol, is lethal. If a single melioidosis organism enters the human bloodstream, death could occur in as little as 7–10 days.

Signs and Symptoms

In nature, both glanders and melioidosis may present as either acute or chronic; acute illness progressing rapidly to death is the more likely outcome of bioterrorism. Glanders enters the body through invasion of the nose, mouth, or eyes, by inhalation into the lungs, or through breaks in the skin. It can then manifest in the form of a local skin infection, or it can enter the bloodstream and spread systemically through all parts of the body. Beware: a local infection and ulcer of the nose could lead to death quite rapidly if it spreads and enters the bloodstream.

The most commonly reported symptoms include high fever, extreme congestion caused by thick mucus, and multiorgan abscesses, predominantly in the lungs, liver and spleen. Other symptoms include swollen glands, lesions, including papules and postules reminiscent of smallpox, jaundice, and pneumonia. The chest x-ray may show pneumonia and lung abnormalities, including massive necrotic lung lesions.

To suspect glanders or melioidosis, look for initial fever of 102°F or higher, headache, muscle pain, night sweats, chest pain, jaundice, sensitivity to light, and diarrhea. In the most dangerous form of the disease, ulcers and bloody nodules form in the nasal cavities, secreting bloody discharge and often causing toxic infection. Bronchitis and pneumonia are hallmarks of both. As infection spreads throughout the body, look for formation of a pus-filled, smallpoxlike rash. Most patients progress rapidly from this stage of the disease to shock and, ultimately, death. For those who remain untreated, mortality is virtually 100% certain within a month of the time symptoms begin. For those who are treated, symptoms—and infection itself—can reappear years to decades later. Mclioidosis, particularly, may lay dormant in the body for years before causing illness. It can also cause chronic metastatic illness and seed the brain, heart, liver, bone, spleen, lymph nodes, and eyes.

How Medical Experts Diagnose Glanders and Melioidosis

While it is possible to diagnose glanders and melioidosis through serology and DNA analysis, such diagnosis must never be the bar for treatment. One reason is that many infected patients test negative on current tests; another is that many patients test positive only when extremely close to death. The best diagnostic clue can come from microscopic study—both these organisms take on a safety-pin appearance when exposed to specific laboratory stains.

Glanders and melioidosis must remain clinical diagnoses if patients hope to survive. Moreover, since the lesions associated with glanders resemble those of smallpox, physicians must also suspect they are dealing with that devastating disease until confirmed otherwise.

Care and Treatment

Treatment guidelines for localized disease include:

- 60–150 days of amoxicillin or clavulanate 60 mg/kg/day in three divided doses for 60–150 days, depending upon severity of disease.
- Tetracycline, 40 mg/kg/day in three divided doses for 60–150 days, depending upon severity of disease.
- TMP/SMX (TMP, 4 mg/kg/day; sulfa, 20 mg/kg/day) in two divided doses for 60–150 days, depending upon severity of disease.

For more severe disease, the U.S. Army recommends combining two of the therapies above for 30 days and then continuing with just one medication for the next 5 to 11 months, depending upon severity of the symptoms.

In the case of systemic disease, you will require intravenous treatment for 2 weeks before changing to the oral antibiotics for 5–11 months, as follows:

- Ceftazidime, 120 mg/kg/day IV in three divided doses and TMP/SMX (TMP, 8 mg/kg/day; sulfa 50, mg/kg/day) IV in four divided doses.

There is no prophylactic treatment currently prescribed for glanders or melioidosis, but Dr. Rega suggests that doctors consider the antibiotic TMP/SMX for this purpose.

What You Need to Know to Survive Glanders and Melioidosis

- If there is an attack in your area, consult with your physician and monitor yourself and your family for fever. If you develop a fever or any type of illness get to a hospital or a designated clinic at once.
- Keep a close lookout for those most susceptible to illness, including the very young, the very old, and the immunocompromised.
- If you are diagnosed with glanders or melioidosis or are determined to be at high risk for exposure, get evaluated for treatment at once. Remember, these diseases are deadly.
- You are talking long-term treatment—1–12 months, depending

upon the severity of symptoms. Because treatment can last for up to a year, some people become noncompliant with treatment over time. Don't let this happen to you, since a lapse in medication could be fatal.

- Report suspected cases of glanders or melioidosis to your local health department. The local health department is responsible for notifying the state health department, the FBI, and local law enforcement. The state health department will notify the CDC.

THE VIRUSES

Viruses are the simplest form of life, consisting merely of a genetic core—RNA- or DNA-based—and a protein coat to surround it. Much smaller than bacteria, which are complete cells that may live alone, viruses are intracellular parasites and lack a system for their own metabolism. Dependent upon the machinery of their host cells for survival, viruses cannot be cultured in the lab. Instead, each virus requires its own special type of host cell to live and multiply—often to the extreme detriment, and even death, of the host.

8

Smallpox

Delivery: Inhalation of aerosol or, alternatively, exposure to a "suicide" carrier.

Symptoms: The sudden appearance of malaise, fevers, vomiting, headache, and backache. After 2–4 days, skin lesions appear and progress uniformly as pus accumulates. Lesions scab in 1–2 weeks. In unvaccinated individuals, variola major, the classical form of smallpox, is fatal in approximately 30% of those who have never been vaccinated.

Timeline: Incubation period from exposure to first symptom is about 12 days.

Can be mistaken for: Chicken pox, varicella, a virus, drug side-effects, impetego, disseminated herpes simplex, and erythema multiforme (an allergic reaction with many different causes that often starts as a red rash on the palms, soles, and back of the hands). While smallpox is not generally similar to any other disease, it may well confound physicians who see the first patients to present with infection. Doctors may be especially prone to confuse smallpox infection in vaccinated individuals with chicken pox.

Treatment: Supportive care is the mainstay of smallpox therapy. No specific antiviral therapy exists. Vaccine may prevent or ameliorate the disease if received shortly after exposure and before symptoms start.

Smallpox in Nature

Smallpox once was humankind's most deadly natural enemy, responsible for killing more people throughout history than any other disease. In fact, smallpox was the single largest cause of human death until vaccination was discovered around 1800, when its use became a standard of health throughout the world.

Today, smallpox, the DNA virus, is considered by most experts to be extinct. Eradication of the microbe, called variola, is one of health care's great achievements in the modern world. In the international effort to rid the world of smallpox, spearheaded by the World Health Organization, workers traveled from continent to continent, chasing down pockets of the disease and vaccinating everyone within a wide radius. The virus, which needs human hosts to survive, was cornered and eliminated.

With smallpox gone from the United States for more than 30 years, mass vaccinations have long since ended. The World Health Organization says the last smallpox death occurred in 1977, and without a disease, vaccination served no further purpose. This means millions of persons now are extremely vulnerable if smallpox is released into the environment.

Smallpox as a Weapon of Biological Terror

Smallpox was first used as a biological weapon during the French and Indian Wars (1754–67), when British forces in North America distributed blankets used by smallpox patients to American Indians aiding the French. The resulting epidemics killed more than 50% of many affected tribes.

The threat of smallpox as a bioweapon was dramatically reduced in 1796, when Edward Jenner showed that an infection caused by cowpox protected against smallpox, laying the intellectual framework for a vaccine. The practice of cowpox inoculation—in other words, vaccination—spread rapidly around the world, diminishing the smallpox threat.

A global campaign, begun in 1967 under the aegis of the World Health Organization, succeeded in eradicating smallpox in 1977. But much to our peril, it was not eradicated in the final sense of the word. Though smallpox no longer infects human populations, the scientists studying it kept a few samples alive in the lab. Today's predicament—and the fear that smallpox could make an appearance as a weapon of biological terror—stems from two small frozen vials of smallpox virus kept under lock and key in the United States and the former Soviet Union. It is now widely accepted as fact that military researchers of the former Soviet Union used part of their supply to manufacture and stockpile tons of weaponized smallpox, possibly exporting their technologies and cultures around the world to the highest bidder when the Soviet Union collapsed.

In the mid-1990s, Russian defector Ken Alibek sent up the alarm when he testified that his laboratory in Koltsovo, the State Research Center of Virology and Biotechnology, had turned its small vial of experimental virus into tons of biological weapon—and had gone so far as to figure out how to launch it on a missile. Alibek also noted that the Soviets had created smallpox hybrids—weapons that combined smallpox and other deadly diseases, including Marburg (an Ebola-like illness), into a single, genetically altered, killer germ.

With the dissolution of the Soviet Union, no one can be sure of the location of all of this deadly pathogen. "It is a very worrisome situation," said Donald A. Henderson, director of the original worldwide eradication effort and now director of the new Office of Public Health Preparedness. Indeed, recent intelligence reports suggest that Soviet scientists are now weaponizing the virus for nations such as Iran, Iraq, Libya, and North Korea. "Many [Russian] scientists are really quite desperate for money," Henderson said recently, adding that there is evidence they have been recruited by "rogue states" and were in a position to smuggle the virus out.

Other reports, meanwhile, indicate that researchers in Australia used genetic engineering to modify a related virus, called mousepox. Ordinary mousepox infects mice and, in its new form, was much deadlier to its hosts—even those who had been immunized.

Could the same be done with smallpox? No one knows.

"As we look at the agents that might be used for biological warfare," Henderson said, "smallpox is at the top of the list."

Of all the biological threats, smallpox has perhaps the greatest potential as a terror weapon because it is so highly contagious, so untreatable, and so deadly. It can be spread to humans through the air, and just a few particles are needed to cause the disease. Initial symptoms include fever and then severe aches and pains. After a few days, a rash appears in the oral cavity and then on the skin, growing into painful pustules the size of peas. Victims become infectious during the first sign of rash as the virus is shed from lesions in the mouth. One victim passes it to another and, as panic sets in, persons who don't realize they are infected flee immediate danger only to spread it further still.

This is particularly relevant for suicide terrorists—imagine how easy it would be to infect oneself and then just walk through a city. A dozen such individuals could create a worldwide pandemic. Dr. Rega notes that while viable, the suicide carrier would be an "impaired weapon" due to his own, increasingly severe disease and therefore, "may not be able to complete his mission." Though he need only to infect a single individual for the mission to be a success.

Such a terrorist might do the most damage by visiting an area of mass transport like an airport or train station, Rega adds. "He would be able to infect people going all over the country, and the CDC would never be able to keep up. It may be that just as we are now inspecting bags and asking people to take off coats and shoes in airports, we will soon have security checking all passengers for fever. Anyone with fever over 100°F wouldn't be allowed on board!"

But in the end, an aerosol rlease of smallpox might be the method of attack. Indeed, the *Journal of the American Medical Association* recently pointed out, "A clandestine aerosol release of smallpox, even if it infected only 50 to 100 persons in the first generation of cases, would rapidly spread in a now highly susceptible population, expanding by a factor of 10 to 20 times or more with each generation of cases. Between the time of an aerosol release of smallpox virus and diagnosis of the first cases, an interval as long as 2 weeks or more is apt to occur."

One way to reduce the risk is to complete the destruction of all remaining smallpox virus, still stored in laboratories in nations around the world. Writing in the journal *Clinical Infectious Diseases* last year, Henderson urged elimination as soon as possible. The stockpiles have been maintained beyond a 1999 deadline for destruction because some researchers argued they would be required to develop new antiviral therapies and improved vaccines, and to anticipate and fend off genetically engineered smallpox weapons that terrorists might engineer in the lab. But Henderson claims these goals are not worth the risk. The research would also "define a whole new array of bioweapons, more awesome than any now known," he states. "And, predictably, these would not be kept secret for very long."

Because smallpox is a virus and not a bacterum, it will not respond to antibiotics. Therefore, it is more difficult to defend against than, say, anthrax or the plague. Nonetheless, from use of electrolyte drinks such as Pedialyte or Gatorade to appropriate quarantine procedures, there are things that can be done in the face of an epidemic to reduce chance of exposure and to increase chance of survival should illness set in.

While vaccination can protect against the disease if provided prior to or up to four days after exposure, as of early 2002, the United States had only enough vaccine for 15 million people—with much of that already allocated for health care workers who will go into stricken areas to treat the sick. Experts say that at least 40 million doses would be required to stanch a regional attack. To fill out the Military stockpile, the Department of Defense has a contract with Dynport Corporation for 300,000 doses. To expand the civilian stockpile, the CDC has contracted with OraVax (renamed Acambis) of Cambridge, Massachusetts, for 40 million doses, with delivery expected by mid-2004.

More recently, Health and Human Services Secretary Tommy G. Thompson announced plans for 250 million additional doses, enough for each and every American. He has expressed the desire to see the stockpiles completed by 2003, but many experts fear the timeline may be overly ambitious, and hope production can be ramped up fast enough to circumvent a smallpox attack.

Signs and Symptoms

Most likely only 10–15% of the U.S. population has residual smallpox immunity based on previous vaccination. These people, if infected, may experience milder forms of infection, but for those not immunized there is no such thing as mild or subclinical disease. Of those who are infected, 25–30% will die.

The timeline for infection with weaponized versions of the bug is as follows: After aerosol exposure, viral organisms travel from the respiratory tract to regional lymph nodes and replicate. Between the time of an aerosol release of smallpox and the emergence of symptoms, there may be an interval of as much as 2 weeks. This is because the average incubation period is 12 to 14 days.

The first signs of the disease are fever (100% of patients), backache (90%), headache (90%), chills (60%), and vomiting (50%). After 2–3 days the patient develops lesions in the oral cavity. It is at this stage that he is most infectious, spreading the virus by cough, sneeze, or vomit. The rash thereafter spreads to palms and soles, face, arms, legs, and torso. A day or two after the external rash appears, it becomes eruptive, blistering on the 4th to 5th day out, and then filling with puss by day 7. The "pustules" are characteristically round, tense, and deeply embedded in the skin; crusts begin to form about the 8th or 9th day, and scabs form by day 14. When the scabs separate perhaps 21 days after symptoms start, pigment-free skin remains, and eventually pitted scars form. Less frequent complications include encephalitis, secondary bacterial infections, conjunctivitis, and blindness.

Smallpox may also present in unconventional fashion. The Center for Bioterrorism points out that there are three variants of the disease, each identified by the features of its rash. "In an outbreak setting," says the center, "these atypical presentations should be considered as smallpox until proven otherwise." Classical smallpox accounts for more than 90% of cases, but you can also be on the lookout for the "flat" variety of rash, which has a velvety appearance and never matures into pustules. More than 95% of patients with a "flat" rash die. There is also the "hemorrhagic" variety, in which the rash is more diffuse and prone to bleeding. This type of smallpox is uniformly fatal.

No matter what form it takes, smallpox would spread rapidly through face-to-face contact, from person-to-person—especially in the beginning when diagnosis may be delayed—it may also spread through infected clothes and bedding. Because oral lesions may be difficult to detect at first, the CDC advises that people must be considered contagious as soon as fever begins. Based on past experience, experts estimate that 30% of those with classic disease will die as a result of massive inflammatory response and overwhelming infection. Individuals who have been vaccinated in the past should be partially immune, and for them, the course of illness is expected to be swifter and less severe. Dr. Rega, meanwhile, points out that, as with anthrax, the actual prognosis for smallpox in the modern healthcare setting is unknown. The death rate could be higher because of all the immunocompromised people in our population, he notes, or it could be lower because of better medical science.

How Medical Professionals Diagnose Smallpox

According to the Center for the Study of Bioterrorism and Emerging Infections, diagnosis in an outbreak setting should be made based on clinical presentation alone.

In theory, the symptoms of smallpox should be easy to diagnose in individuals who have not been vaccinated. The small, pus-filled skin lesions are unlike symptoms associated with any other disease. But in practice, physicians are simply unfamiliar with the disease—most, in fact, have never seen it. They may therefore become confused, and can have special difficulty in detecting rarer, variant forms of the illness in which the skin lesions are flat, or bleed. Among the conditions that inexperienced physicians may mistake for smallpox are varicella, a virus, drug side-effects, impetego, disseminated herpes simplex, and erythema multiforme (an allergic reaction with many different causes that often starts as a red rash on the palms, soles, and back of the hands). It can spread to the trunk, face, and mouth in severe cases. While smallpox is not generally similar to any other disease, it may well confound physicians who see the first patients to present with infection. Smallpox infection in vaccinated individuals may sometimes be confused with chicken pox.

Despite their similarities, the difference between smallpox and chicken pox is vast. Initial symptoms of headache, fever, and backache are absent or mild in chicken pox. Lesions, while intensely itchy, are superficial, concentrating largely on the trunk while uncommon on palms and soles. Chicken pox lesions develop in less than 24 hours, and the illness lasts less than a week. Smallpox lesions, by contrast, begin in the mouth and then spread to the face and extremities, where they remain more concentrated, before spreading to the legs and torso. Notably the palms and soles are not spared and most of the lesions in any given area are in the same stage of development (vesicles, pustules, or scabs). In the case of chicken pox, each new area has lesions in different stages of maturation. Smallpox can now also be confirmed by DNA analysis through rapid polymerase chain reaction (PCR) tests at reference laboratories.

Care and Treatment

There is no proven treatment for full-blown smallpox at this time, and it goes without saying that the United States is dangerously unprepared. No one born after the mid-1970s has been vaccinated—why bother when the disease is gone? And since full immunity lasts for only about 10 years, no one is completely safe. At least one generation of Americans has no protection at all, and another generation has just waning protection.

Once the eradication was complete, the United States stopped making the vaccine, so all that's left are 15 million doses, stored in a freezer housed in a Wyeth-Ayerst warehouse in Lancaster County, Pennsylvania. Experts say at least 40 million doses would be needed to protect against a possible regional attack. While the United States plans to produce and stockpile enough vaccine for each citizen, production lines have yet to launch.

Once production is fired up, the vaccine would mitigate symptoms in the exposed—as long as it was dispensed within 3 or 4 days of exposure. You can tell your vaccination has been successful—that it has exposed you to the mild infection that will enable immunity—if you experience tenderness, swelling, and a pustular lesion at the inoculation site as well as fever, and swollen nodes in the armpit. Experts say such a reaction means that the vaccine "took." If you do not experience this reaction, report it to your doctor so that you can be evaluated for receipt of another dose.

As with many vaccines, there can be serious, even lethal, outcomes to smallpox vaccination; that is why vaccination was suspended after eradication of the disease. Under ordinary circumstances, certain groups would be automatically advised against vaccination, but under epidemic circumstances such individuals will have to weigh the risk of vaccination against the very real risk of disease.

Among those especially prone to complications from smallpox vaccination, according to the CDC and the *Journal of the American Medical Association,* are:

- Anyone with or ever diagnosed as having an eruptive, acute or chronic skin condition like eczema, shingles or impetigo.
- Patients with leukemia, lymphoma, or any kind of malignancy, as well as those receiving cancer treatment.

- HIV patients or anyone with hereditary immune deficiency disorder.
- Pregnant women.
- Those with serious or life-threatening allergies to antibiotics like polymixin B, streptomycin, tetracycline, or neomycin.

Though especially prevalent in these groups, adverse reactions may strike anyone. Their nature and frequency were measured in a 10-state survey of smallpox vaccinees in 1968. In order of occurrence, smallpox vaccine adverse reactions include:

- Inadvertent vaccination, where vaccine gets into the eyes or other inappropriate area. Occurred in 529.2 of every million cases. (Often, irrigating the inappropriately exposed area will prevent a problem.)
- Generalized vaccinia, which is a rash all over the body 6–9 days after vaccination. Affects 241.5 of every million vaccinees.
- Eczema vaccinatum, a form of eczema that is usually mild but fatal in rare instances. Occurs in 38.5 of every million vaccinees.
- Post-vaccinal encephalitis. Just about the worst side effect of smallpox vaccination aside from death, this occurs in 12.3 out of every million vaccinees. On the whole, 25% of those with this reaction suffer permanent neurological damage, and another 15–25% succumb.
- Progressive vaccinia, in which vaccination site widens and surrounding tissue dies. Impacts 1.5 of every million vaccinees.

In all these instances, except for cases of encephalitis, individuals can often be successfully treated with another therapy called vaccinia-immune globulin, or VIG. Used to improve the outcome of smallpox with or without vaccine, VIG, under epidemic conditions, would be reserved for treating of those who have reacted badly to vaccine. Made from the plasma of vaccinated individuals, VIG is available in the United States from the Drug Service of the CDC. The U.S. Army maintains a supply for its own use. (Dose for prophylaxis or treatment is 0.6 ml/kg, administered intramuscularly. Administration immediately after or within the first 24 hours of exposure would provide the highest level of protection, especially in unvaccinated persons.)

VIG does not work for post-vaccine encephalitis, which remains the most disturbing consequence of any national vaccination campaign. There is currently no treatment for those who react to smallpox vaccination in this particular way.

For these reasons, smallpox vaccination cannot be undertaken lightly. Nonetheless, according to the CDC, under circumstances of face-to-face contact, the risk of developing smallpox, even for those more prone to complication, is greater than the risk of the complication itself.

Aside from vaccine and VIG, no drugs have been proven to work for those infected with smallpox. But test tube evidence suggests that antiviral medications, including adefovir, dipivoxil, cidofovir, and ribavirin, have significant in vitro antiviral activity against poxviruses. While the efficacy of these drugs as therapeutic agents for smallpox is currently uncertain, cidofovir is FDA-licensed and shows the most promise in animal models. According to the Center for the Study of Bioterrorism, research shows these antiviral agents may be most effective if taken no more than a day or two after an individual has been exposed.

Antibiotics may also be of use in treating secondary infections that accompany smallpox. If you happen to have some personal supplies of antibiotic around the house, however, these must never be used prophylactically, in the general expectation of an attack, or in the presence of smallpox itself. The particular coinfection must be diagnosed specifically by a physician. If you take the wrong antibiotic, or if you take an antibiotic when you don't need it, you could be doing damage and perhaps even literally breeding resistant bacterial strains.

As with cholera, smallpox patients may become dehydrated. Use guidelines in the cholera chapter to check for dehydration status, and compensate with electrolyte solutions like oral rehydrating solution, Pedialyte or Gatorade. Make sure that infants receive only Pedialyte, since water under conditions of dehydration can cause seizure.

Due to the risk of secondary infection, the smallpox patient will have a better chance of making it through if treated at home. But this poses great risk to the caretaker, who has contact with the patient and can therefore come down with the disease. Indeed, the rate of secondary infection among susceptible household contacts ranges from 38–88%. If you plan to be a caretaker, you should make every effort to obtain vaccination. But in the immediate aftermath of a bioterrorist attack, and in the wake of an epidemic, this may not be possible. The next best thing you can do is take extreme precaution against getting sick.

Make sure the patient has a separate room and, if possible, a separate bathroom. Be sure both you and your patients have disposable HEPA masks, and that you wear them whenever coming into contact with each other. Bag or incinerate all disposable items that have been in contact with the patient. Spray the bag with Lysol or an equivalent disinfectant before taking it out to incinerate. As to sheets, linens, and clothes, you may wash them in very hot water with bleach, or you may bag and incinerate them. Don protective gear such as a disposable surgical gown, mask, and gloves; wash the floors, walls, and furniture of the patient's room with Lysol. When cleaning the patient, be extremely careful not to break any lesions, thus exposing yourself to pus. Your best bet in cleaning the patient is plain, soapy water. Do not use lotions or salves. If at all possible, have a newly vaccinated family member care for the ill. If this is not possible, it is better for the caretaker to have had a vaccination, even 30 years previous, than to call upon a caretaker who has had no vaccination at all.

Given the enormity of the tragedy that a smallpox attack might auger, the powers-that-be will not only treat the immediately infected and those in contact with them, but also do what they can to prevent spread of the disease. In this effort, the CDC will function not just as a health agency, but also as an arm of the military.

It only stands to reason that to protect the rest of society, smallpox patients and anyone in contact with them will have to be isolated from others. Isolation, says Dr. Rega, is defined as the separation of a person or group of persons from other people to prevent spread of infection. Beware that if an outbreak occurs, the CDC plans to assign citizens of threatened areas to one of three zones:

1. Type C (Contagious facility) for known or presumed infected pox people. Should be a special area away from other buildings and people that can give best medical care to patients. All who enter must be vaccinated first.
2. Type X for febrile contacts who do not have a rash. May be a motel, hotel, or dorm. Patients will be monitored for the disease.
3. Type R (Residential facility) for asymptomatic contacts such as household members of those with smallpox. These individuals

will be able to live at home and go about their usual routine. They will be prevented from going 20 miles beyond the town line and will be asked to check their temperature twice daily. These individuals should be vaccinated, if at all possible.

People assigned to "Type R" facilities will be asked to remain under active surveillance for 18 days after their last contact with a pox case or 14 days after successful vaccination. They may go about normal activities within their city of residence, except for checking their temperature twice daily. If temperature is greater than 101°F twice in a row, or if the individual develops a rash, he will be expected to call public health authorities and stay indoors until someone comes.

In addition to isolation, the government may enforce conditions of quarantine with the help of military personnel or the National Guard. While isolation generally refers to individual patients, quarantine is population-wide. While isolation is generally a medical action, quarantine is also a legal one.

Quarantine laws are generally the responsibility of the states but those laws are old and we do not know if they can stand up to constitutional review. In the case of a smallpox attack, if states are unable to enforce a quarantine, the federal government, under the auspices of an agency like the CDC, will step in. Representatives would be empowered to close buildings, take control of hospitals, order and enforce quarantine, mandate medical exams, enforce treatment like vaccination, and ration supplies, including medication and food.

Some 30 years ago, in an era of peace, smallpox was finally brought under control worldwide through what experts call "ring vaccination." In this approach, confirmed and suspected cases are traced and isolated while all those in contact with these individuals are observed. Potential cases and their contacts are vaccinated, essentially forming a "ring" around the infected area. The ring of vaccination prevents the virus from leaping outside the zone of infection, and eventually the disease is contained.

During any smallpox outbreak, those within the ring of vaccination would include individuals exposed during the initial release at ground zero, if that can be determined, as well as anyone with symptoms of the disease; "contacts," defined as anyone who has come within 6 feet of the exposed or infected after the attack; household members of the infected and exposed; and household members of contacts. You can see how quickly this "ring" would expand to encompass virtually everyone in a city under siege.

Vaccinees would also include anyone directly involved in patient care, patient evaluation, or patient transportation. In this group are doctors, nurses, and hospital aides or workers of any kind; lab personnel; and law enforcement or military staff (who may be charged with preventing citizens from leaving or entering the "ring of vaccination," and who would have to "enforce" treatment in those who refused).

The ultimate treatment for smallpox may be frightening, indeed. The government may have to enforce vaccination of the exposed to prevent spread of the disease, and it may have to enforce quarantine of those who refuse vaccination or become ill. The vision of soldiers with guns preventing people from entering or leaving a stricken area or an entire city seems decidedly un-American. Yet it is the "treatment" that may, by necessity, be front and center in containing disease.

What You Need to Know to Survive an Attack of Smallpox

- Smallpox spreads easily via respiratory droplets generated in ordinary talking and breathing.
- All suspected cases of smallpox should be isolated immediately, and they should remain isolated until all scabs separate from the body.
- It is preferable to spend this period of isolation at home instead of at a hospital, if possible, because of the high risk of secondary bacterial infection in an institutional setting.
- Anyone who has been in contact with an infected individual should be identified, vaccinated, and monitored twice a day for development of fever, which may indicate the onset of smallpox. Monitoring should continue for 17 days after the contact has taken place, or for 14 days after vaccination.
- You can tell your vaccination has been successful—that it has exposed you to the mild infection that will enable immunity—if you experience tenderness, swelling, and a pustular lesion at the inocu-

lation site as well as fever, and swollen nodes in the armpit. Experts say such a reaction means that the vaccine "took." If you do not experience this reaction, report it to your doctor so that you can be evaluated for receipt of another dose.

- Smallpox vaccine can cause permanent neurological damage or even death in a small percent of recipients. HIV patients, cancer patients, pregnant women, and those with skin disease are especially at risk. But the CDC says that those who have been exposed to smallpox are at greater risk for smallpox than side effects, even if they are part of a high-risk group.

- For those never vaccinated, 25–40% will contract smallpox upon contact with an infected individual. The form and the severity of smallpox that emerges will be unaffected by the form or severity of disease in the individual who is sick.

- If you are caring for a loved one with smallpox, you must wear proper respiratory protection, including a mask, along with gown and gloves.

- The sickroom should be cleaned with disinfectant regularly. You may use either quaternary ammonia or bleach.

- Smallpox virus can live for extended periods in clothing and bed linens. Linens used by infected or exposed individuals should be washed in hot water with bleach and dried at high temperature, or simply discarded.

- Make sure that dehydrated infants receive only Pedialyte, since water under conditions of dehydration can cause them to experience seizure.

- Be sure to keep plenty of fluid, especially electrolyte, on hand, since smallpox patients may become dehydrated.

- Smallpox victims may become even sicker as the result of secondary bacterial infections. These infections require antibiotics, but you should strive for a specific diagnosis from a physician before any antibiotic treatment is rendered, lest the medication make the patient sicker than before.

- In the event of an attack or epidemic, the government may step in to enforce isolation and quarantine under military jurisdiction, and may even enforce vaccination in the stricken area as well as surrounding areas to prevent the disease from spreading.

- Report suspected cases or suspected intentional release of smallpox to your local health department. The local health department is responsible for notifying the state health department, the FBI, and local law enforcement. The state health department will notify the CDC.

- Bodies of deceased victims should be cremated whenever possible.

9

The Viral Hemorrhagic Fevers:

Ebola, Marburg, Lassa, Junin, Yellow Fever, Dengue, Rift Valley Fever, Crimean-Congo Fever, and Hantavirus

Delivery: Inhalation of aerosol.

Symptoms: Marked fever, fatigue, dizziness, muscle aches, loss of strength, and exhaustion. Patients with severe cases of VHF often show signs of bleeding under the skin, in internal organs, or from body orifices like the mouth, eyes, or ears. However, although they may bleed from many sites around the body, patients rarely die because of blood loss. Severely ill patients may also show shock, nervous system malfunction, coma, delirium, and seizures. Some types of VHF are associated with renal (kidney) failure.

Timeline: Incubation period from exposure to appearance of symptoms varies from 4 to 35 days, depending upon the particular virus. Some specifics include yellow fever, 3–6 days; Rift Valley fever, 2–5 days; Ebola, 2–21 days; dengue, 13–15 days; Marburg, 7–15 days; Hanta, up to 35 days.

Can be mistaken for: Malaria, typhoid fever, rickettsial infections, leptospirosis, relapsing fever, hepatitis, leukemia, to name a few diseases that may be confused with VHF.

Treatment: Depending upon the specific VHF, may respond to treatment with antiviral medications, including ribavirin, and can be prevented by vaccine.

Viral Hemorrhagic Fevers in Nature

In September 2000, 38-year-old Rose Abello abruptly developed a fever, started bleeding from every orifice in her body, and died. In her small Uganda town, where many die young, people at first felt grief, but no alarm. Relatives simply washed away the blood as she lay dying, and prepared her body for burial when she was gone. As was the custom, others inherited her clothes. But when her 2-year-old daughter died of the same symptoms the next day, followed by her 13-year-old daughter and then her husband, age 42, relatives and neighbors grew concerned. With good reason: the cause was soon identified as Ebola, one of the deadliest viruses known. Of unknown origin, it spread like wildfire from person to person through contact with bodily fluids and the victims' clothes. Alarm was warranted: a month after the first symptom appeared, 51 people were dead and 139 had been infected by the disease.

The Ebola outbreak in Uganda followed others, notably in Zaire (now Congo), where the disease was first identified some 25 years ago, killing 245. Back then, quarantine procedures contained the infection, samples of which were frozen for posterity and stored at CDC headquarters in Atlanta, Georgia.

It took 20 years for Ebola to resurface in Zaire, this time striking staff and patients at a small community hospital in the city of Kikwit and spreading to dozens of villagers nearby. Again, containment procedures were swift. A CDC SWAT team converged on the region. Wearing protective masks and other garb, investigators went door to door searching for those with symptoms, and armed soldiers prevented anyone from leaving or entering the city until the situation was under control. CDC investigators eventually traced the infection first to a nurse and then to one of her patients. That individual, called "patient zero," was a charcoal worker whose job sent him into the rain forest. Although they had no evidence, scientists theorized he was probably infected by an Ebola-carrying animal, possibly a bat.

Ebola, one of the new "hot viruses" causing so much alarm these days, kills up to 90% of its victims. Like other such diseases, it is thought to emerge when humans have contact with arthropods and other animals inhabiting the tropical rain forest. If not stopped aggressively, say experts, such infections might spread around the world. In West Africa, for example, Lassa virus infects 100,000 to 300,000 people per year, killing more than 5,000 annually. It's transmitted by a rodent called the multimammate rat, found in the savannas and forests of West, Central, and East Africa. And in the United States the hantavirus, a microbe carried by the deer mouse, has infected a total of 250 people. The virus drowns its victims by causing the lungs to fill up with fluid.

According to Thomas V. Inglesby, a physician with the Johns Hopkins University Center for Civilian Biodefense Studies, Ebola and Lassa are two of the viral hemorrhagic fevers (VHFs), caused by a variety of viruses in four major families—arenaviruses, flaviviruses, bunyaviruses, and filoviruses. While VHF organisms are diverse, they have at least two things in common: they are RNA viruses, with a genetic core made of ribonucleic acid, and they cause severe illness characterized foremost by fever and internal bleeding.

The CDC says VHFs have the following in common:

- They are all RNA viruses, and all are enveloped, or covered, in a lipid (fatty) coating.
- Their survival is dependent on an animal or insect host, called the natural reservoir.
- The viruses are geographically restricted to the areas where their host species live.
- Humans are not the natural reservoir for any of these viruses. Humans are infected when they come into contact with infected hosts. However, with some viruses, after the accidental transmission from the host, humans can transmit the virus to one another.
- Human cases or outbreaks of hemorrhagic fevers caused by these viruses occur sporadically and irregularly.
- The occurrence of outbreaks cannot be easily predicted.
- With a few noteworthy exceptions, there is no cure or established drug treatment for VHFs.

No matter what form of VHF under discussion, the course of the disease—although not the timeframe—is generally the same. A poor or delayed immune response enables viral organisms to multiply rapidly. With special affinity for the vascular system, these microbes prevent blood from coagulating and cause increased permeability of blood vessels. The result is that blood literally seeps through capillaries, at first causing flushing, blood shot eyes, and bloody diarrhea. But this is just the beginning. Blood eventually seeps through mucosal tissue in areas such as the nose and mouth, so that the VHF patient hemorrhages through all orifices. In the end, internal organs seem to literally liquefy as the victim bleeds to death from the inside. As the patient melts away, multisystem organ failure may cause pulmonary, neurologic, or any number of other symptoms before ending in circulatory collapse, shock, and death.

Despite the similar *modus operandi,* these viruses differ widely, indeed. In nature, the means of transmission differs from virus to virus, Inglesby says. Biting insects cause dengue and Rift Valley fever or Crimean-Congo hemorrhagic fever, for instance, while Lassa fever results from inhalation of aerosols associated with rodent excrement. For Ebola and Marburg, meanwhile, the route remains unknown. Some of these diseases, such as dengue, can be widespread, while others, such as Ebola and Marburg (named after the German town where it was discovered in 1967), are rare and found in few locations worldwide. Fatality rates vary greatly. For dengue, the mortality rate may be as low as 1%. But the 1976 Ebola epidemic in Zaire had a fatality rate of 92%.

While a true accounting of these viruses might require a textbook, the fourth edition of the U.S. Army's *Medical Management of Biological Casualties Handbook* has done an admirable job of differentiating between them, in brief, through a description of four broad groups:

Arenaviruses Argentine hemorrhagic fever (AHF), caused by the Junin virus, was first described in 1955 in corn harvesters. Argentina sees from 300 to 600 cases per year. Bolivian, Brazilian, and Venezuelan hemorrhagic fevers, meanwhile, are caused by the related Machupo, Guanarito, and Sabia viruses. Lassa virus causes disease in West Africa. These viruses are transmitted from rodents to humans by the inhalation of dusts contaminated with rodent excreta.

Bunyaviruses Crimean-Congo hemorrhagic fever (CCHF) is a tick-borne disease that occurs in the Crimea and in parts of Africa, Europe, and Asia. It can also be spread by contact with infected animals, and in health care settings. Rift Valley fever (RVF) is a mosquito-borne disease that occurs in Africa. The hantaviruses are rodent-borne viruses with a wide geographic distribution. Hantaan and closely related viruses cause hemorrhagic fever with renal syndrome (HFRS; also known as Korean hemorrhagic fever or epidemic hemorrhagic fever). These viruses were described prior to World War II in Manchuria along the

Amur River, among United Nations troops during the Korean conflict, and subsequently in Japan, China, and the Russian Far East. Severe disease also occurs in some Balkan states, including Bosnia, Serbia, and Greece. In addition, newly described hantaviruses cause hantavirus pulmonary syndrome (HPS) in the Americas. The hantaviruses are transmitted to humans by the inhalation of dust contaminated with rodent waste.

Filoviruses   Ebola hemorrhagic fever is a severe, often-fatal disease in humans and nonhuman primates (monkeys and chimpanzees) that has appeared sporadically since its initial recognition in 1976, according to the CDC. The disease is caused by infection with Ebola virus, named after a river in the Democratic Republic of the Congo (formerly Zaire) in Africa, where it was first recognized. The virus is one of two members of a family of RNA viruses called the Filoviridae. Three of the four species of Ebola virus identified so far have caused disease in humans: Ebola-Zaire, Ebola-Sudan, and Ebola-Ivory Coast (all named for nations where outbreaks occurred). The fourth species, Ebola-Reston, has caused disease in nonhuman primates, but not in humans. Marburg fever epidemics have occurred on six occasions: five times in Africa, and once in Europe. The first recognized outbreak occurred in Marburg, Germany, and in Yugoslavia, among people exposed to African green monkeys, and resulted in 31 cases and 7 deaths. Filoviruses can be spread from human to human by direct contact with infected blood, secretions, organs, or semen.

Flaviviruses   Yellow fever and dengue, the two most prominent diseases of this group, are spread by mosquitoes. Other flaviviruses are spread by ticks, including the agents of Kyanasur Forest disease in India and Omsk hemorrhagic fever in Siberia.

VHF as a Weapon of Biological Terror

All of the VHF agents (except for dengue virus) are infectious by aerosol in the laboratory. Because they are maintained in animal reservoirs, they are also available around the globe. In view of their aerosol infectivity, their availability, and their lethality, viral hemorrhagic fevers make potent candidates for weapons of biological war.

RECOGNIZED VIRAL HEMORRHAGIC FEVERS OF HUMANS

Virus Family Genus	Disease (Virus)	Natural Distribution	Source of Human Infection Usual	Less Likely	Incubation (Days)
Arenaviridae *Arenavirus*	Lassa fever	Africa	Rodent	Hospital	5–16
	Argentine HF (Junin)	South America	Rodent	Hospital	7–14
	Bolivian HF (Machupo)	South America	Rodent	Hospital	9–15
	Brazilian HF (Sabia)	South America	Rodent	Hospital	7–14
	Venezuelan HF (Guanarito)	South America	Rodent	Hospital	7–14
Bunyaviridae *Phlebovirus*	Rift Valley fever	Africa	Mosquito	Slaughter of domestic animal	2–5
Nairovirus	Crimean-Congo HF	Europe, Asia, Africa	Tick	Slaughter of domestic animal; Hospital	3–12
Hantavirus	Hantaan and related viruses	Asia, Europe; possibly worldwide	Rodent		9–35
Filoviridae *Filovirus*	Marburg and Ebola	Africa	Unknown	Hospital	3–16
Flaviviridae *Flavivirus* (Mosquito-borne)	Yellow fever	Tropical Africa, South America	Mosquito		3–6
	Dengue	Asia, Americas, Africa	Mosquito		Unknown for dengue HF, but 3–5 for uncomplicated dengue
(Tick-borne)	Kyasanur Forest disease	India	Tick		3–8
	Omsk	Russia	Tick	Muskrats, contaminated water	3–8

Source: U.S. Army Medical Research Institute of Infectious Diseases.

Should a viral hemorrhagic fever become an agent of terrorism, moreover, U.S. health care providers would have scant experience as they tried to diagnose the disease and care for the ill. In fact, there is just one VHF, yellow fever, that Western physicians have much experience with at all.

Terrorists—even before they were called that—have long recognized the potential of yellow fever to wreak havoc in war. During the Civil War, Confederate spies based in Canada even tried to press their cause by distributing the clothing of yellow fever victims through the cities of the North. The plan didn't work, in large part because yellow fever cannot be transmitted by clothes.

It was just over a century ago that the U.S. Army Yellow Fever Commission published its classic experiments showing this scourge of the battlefield was not, as previously assumed, transmitted from person to person or via clothing but, rather, by mosquitoes. Calling yellow fever "the original hemorrhagic fever," vaccine researcher Thomas P. Monath of the Massachusetts biotechnology company, Acambis, recently observed that while Ebola makes the headlines, yellow fever is "a much more important medical problem." Even today there are more than 200,000 cases a year with a case-fatality rate of 20–50%.

Yellow fever originated in Africa in the 1500s and came to America with the slave trade. Experts estimate there were some 135 epidemics in the United States from 1668 through 1893, hitting the southern and eastern seaboard as far north as Boston. In 1793, a yellow fever epidemic killed a tenth of the residents in Philadelphia. Another epidemic in 1878 killed 20,000 people in the Mississippi Valley.

For centuries no one knew what caused the disease, though theories abounded—from the idea of some vague "effluvium" spreading person to person to the notion of transmission through clothing and bed linens to the suggestion that mosquitoes were involved. The disease continued to cause panic, and to be misunderstood, until 1900, in the midst of the Spanish-American War and U.S. occupation of Cuba. With hundreds of American soldiers on Cuban soil succumbing to yellow fever, the Army's surgeon general, George Miller Sternberg, sent a board to investigate.

The Yellow Fever Commission, headed by Major Walter Reed, conducted their experiments on themselves and military volunteers. In one test, volunteers spent several weeks sleeping on bed linen that had been soiled with vomit, blood, urine, and feces from yellow fever patients. None of the volunteers fell ill. In another test, a building was divided into two chambers separated by a fine metal screen. On one side of the screen, volunteers lived in quarters infested with mosquitoes that had fed on yellow fever patients, and these volunteers fell ill; those on the other side of the screen breathed the same air as the first group but were protected from the mosquitoes. They did not come down with the disease.

After the results were published in the *Journal of the American Medical Association* in 1901, Cuba drained its marshes, screened water containers, and treated standing water with kerosene to kill mosquito larvae. Although Havana had reported at least one case of yellow fever a day since 1762, in 90 days the disease was gone.

But the ability to rid a city of mosquitoes is unlikely to help fight weaponized yellow fever, which, like most other VHFs explored as tools of terror and attack, can be rendered in aerosol form. The United States, for instance, weaponized yellow fever in one of the earliest biowarfare efforts of modern times.

The VHFs, in fact, make excellent candidates for the most catastrophic scenarios in any terrorist war. According to Peter Jahrling, Ph.D., senior research scientist at the U.S. Army Medical Research Institute of Infectious Diseases in Fort Detrick, Maryland, "The VHF agents are all highly infectious via the aerosol route, and most are quite stable as respirable aerosols. This means that they satisfy at least one criterion for being weaponized, and some clearly have the potential to be biological warfare threats. Most of these agents replicate in cell culture to concentrations sufficiently high to produce a small terrorist weapon, one suitable for introducing lethal doses of virus into the air intake of an airplane or office building. Some replicate to even higher concentrations, with obvious potential ramifications."

Yellow fever is unlikely to be the only VHF yet weaponized. It is well known in the intelligence community, for instance, that the Soviets sent people to Africa looking for Ebola and Marburg. Ken Alibek, former chief scientist of the Soviet bioweapons program before defecting to the West, reports that the Soviets were successful in weaponizing these germs.

Alibek's description of the Soviets' work resulting in a stable Marburg weapon is especially notable. The Soviets had been working with the virus for about a decade, Alibek explains, when in 1988, Nikolai Ustinov, leader of the Marburg research, accidentally injected the virus into his thumb. Despite great effort, it was impossible to save Ustinov, but the Soviet bioweaponeers made sure he did not die in vain. "A virus grown in laboratory conditions is liable to become more virulent when it passes through the live incubator of a human or animal body," clarifies Alibek. It was not unexpected, therefore, when the virus extracted from Ustinov upon autopsy turned out to be "much more powerful and stable" than the strain that had infected him in the first place. It was Marburg Variant U (for Ustinov) that the Soviet Ministry of Defense finally approved as part of its biological arsenal in 1990. Ustinov himself, Alibek wrote, would have applauded the result.

South Africa, meanwhile, is said to have had a bioweapons arsenal including Ebola and Marburg (as well as the AIDS virus) before the fall of apartheid. Western intelligence learned that after white rule ended in 1994, Muammar Qadaffi of Libya tried to hire South African scientists for his nation's efforts in germ warfare. The Russians are known to have strains not just of Ebola and Marburg, but also of Lassa fever, in storage still.

Genetic engineering, meanwhile, brings new meaning to the terror that hemorrhagic fevers can cause. Ken Alibek has warned of a sleight of hand the Soviets devised, involving incorporation of Ebola or Marburg genes into a smallpox virus body, creating a hybrid biological weapon that could bring more destruction—as if that were even imaginable—than either germ alone. Indeed, while smallpox is highly infectious, once it was recognized, it could be controlled by vaccine so that those exposed would not succumb. Ebola is not as infectious, but it is more lethal, and there is no known treatment or cure.

The first step for the Soviets, Alibek explains, was to "explore the genome of the smallpox virus as fully as possible, to facilitate genetic engineering operations with it and to enable an accurate comparison with related viruses." The work, he goes on, had the eventual goal of "manipulating smallpox virulence factors and inserting genes of other viruses into smallpox to create chimera viruses [organisms composed of genetic material from two or more viruses]. The purpose of creating chimera viruses was to design new organisms which would have a synergistic effect and/or evade current vaccines or treatments." To fool the West, the Soviets worked largely with vaccinia (cowpox) virus, an organism so genetically similar to smallpox it can be used as a model in the lab. Alibek explains that "special research was done to find a spot in the vaccinia genome into which foreign genes could be inserted without disrupting viral virulence. Again, this research work was presented as essential for the development of new vaccines by inserting foreign genes into vaccinia. However, for human vaccines based on vaccinia virus, virulence would not be important. On the other hand, if this research were being conducted for the eventual purpose of inserting foreign genes into smallpox for biological weapons purposes, preserving virulence would indeed be important."

It seems plausible to many that Russian scientists have continued this line of research, and in 1998 the Clinton administration explored the possible outcome of a "double whammy" in a scenario for top aides. In the practice exercise, terrorists released their biological weapon along the U.S.-Mexican border, in California and the Southwest. The emerging epidemic was easily diagnosed as smallpox, and the population was vaccinated for protection, apparently limiting the spread of infection. But a few weeks later, after the spread of smallpox had presumably been controlled, genes from the second infection—Marburg virus—kicked into play. This secondary infection, without treatment or cure, was almost impossible to halt.

Signs and Symptoms

As their name suggests, viral hemorrhagic fevers are characterized by fever and bleeding. Early symptoms include fever, headache, fatigue, abdominal pain, muscle aches—much like the flu. Because these viruses target capillaries and the vascular system, the second tier of symptoms could include bloody diarrhea, bleeding gums, rash, red or purplish discoloration on the skin, and general edema (swelling). Eventually, as the various organs become compromised, the patient will show neurological symptoms, ranging from rage to disorientation, and then finally, shock and death.

It is beyond the scope of this book to differentiate among some 20 related VHFs, many of which are unrelated from an evolutionary point of view. Instead, we describe in greater detail the VHFs the CDC says present the most likelihood of weaponization, and the greatest level of risk. These include the filoviruses (Ebola and Marburg) and the arenaviruses (Lassa and Junin).

How to Recognize Ebola and Marburg

- Initial symptom constellation including fever, headache, muscular pain, abdominal pain, and diarrhea.
- Chest pain, cough, pharyngitis, photophobia, and conjunctivitis.
- Jaundice.
- About 5 days after onset, a rash on the trunk of the body.
- Central nervous system symptoms, including psychosis, delirium, coma, and seizures.
- As the disease progresses, bleeding symptoms may include nosebleed, bloody diarrhea, and facial flushing.
- Shock and multiple organ failure by the second week of illness.
- The case-fatality rate for Marburg virus is about 25%; for the various strains of Ebola virus it ranges from 50 to 90%.

How to Recognize Lassa Virus

- Indigenous cases in West Africa often are subclinical or involve only mild symptoms.
- Illness presents with fever and a variety of other symptoms, including chest pain, cough, abdominal pain, vomiting, diarrhea, and conjunctivitis.
- Central nervous system involvement may occur (including encephalitis, encephalopathy, and meningeal signs).
- Symptoms associated with abnormal bleeding occur in about 20% of patients.
- Complications include spontaneous abortion among pregnant women and eighth cranial nerve deafness.
- The overall case-fatality rate is low (about 1%), but among hospitalized patients the rate is about 20%.

How to Recognize Junin and Other South American Hemorrhagic Fever Viruses

- Onset is insidious, with fever, muscle pain, and headache.
- Illness progresses to either a vascular syndrome (hemorrhagic

complications and capillary leak syndrome) or a neurologic syndrome (cerebellar signs and seizures).
- Acute illness lasts several weeks, and recovery may be prolonged.
- The case-fatality rate is 15 to 30%.

For the true diagnosticians, other distinguishing characteristics follow:

- Jaundice is seen only in yellow fever and in Rift Valley, Crimean-Congo, Marburg, and Ebola hemorrhage fevers.
- Marburg and Ebola victims experience a swelling of the palate along with flulike symptoms in the initial states of the disease. Some 5–6 days later they develop pinhead-sized eruptions which, within 24 hours, turn into larger, often flatter, hemorrhaging lesions.
- Kyanasur Forest disease and Omsk hemorrhagic fever are notable for pulmonary involvement and central nervous system symptoms.
- Lassa fever can cause severe edema due to capillary leak, but hemorrhage is uncommon, while hemorrhage is commonly caused by the South American arenaviruses.
- Severe hemorrhage is common in Crimean-Congo hemorrhagic fever.
- Hearing loss is common among Lassa fever survivors.
- Hantavirus victims will manifest tiny, purple and red eruptions on neck, arms, and trunk. Also: flushed skin, bleeding gums and eyes.

How Medical Professionals Diagnose the Viral Hemorrhagic Fevers

Definite diagnosis of VHF comes from laboratory testing, including detection of viral antigens or an antibody response to the virus in the blood. According to the U.S. Army's *Medical Management of Biological Casualties Handbook*, diagnosis should ideally start with a detailed travel history to show possibility of having contracted the disease. Patients with arenavirus or hantavirus infections often recall having seen rodents during the presumed incubation period, but since the viruses are spread to man by aerosolized excreta or environmental contamination, actual contact with the reservoir is not necessary.

Large mosquito populations are common during Rift Valley fever or flavivirus transmission, but a history of mosquito bite is too common to be of diagnostic importance, whereas tick bites or hospital exposure are of some significance in suspecting Crimean-Congo HF. Large numbers of people presenting with VHF manifestations in the same geographic area over a short time period should lead treating medical care providers to suspect either a natural outbreak in an endemic setting or possibly a biowarfare attack, particularly if this type of disease does not occur naturally in the local area.

VHF should be suspected in any patient presenting with high fever and evidence of damage or imbalance involving bleeding and the flow of blood. Easy bleeding, including nosebleeds, flushing of face and chest, and edema may all be diagnostic signs.

Dr. Paul Rega, author of *Bio-Terry: A Stat Manual to Identify and Treat Diseases of Biological Terrorism* (the ultimate guide for hospital emergency departments), notes that physicians may also seek other clues in the blood: a decrease in the number of white blood cells, a decrease in the absolute number of platelets, elevated liver enzymes, and abnormal blood clotting times may support other evidence that a viral hemorrhagic fever is, in fact, in play.

Remember, although laboratory tests are required for an absolute diagnosis, in the event of a catastrophic biological attack where VHF has been proved in at least some individuals, you will not have time to wait for the return of test results. Diagnosis by virus cultivation and identification will require 3 to 10 days or longer, by which time the infected individual may have died.

Care and Treatment

The best place for a patient with viral hemorrhagic fever is the hospital, under the care of medical professionals. In contained situations where just a few are ill, this should be easily achieved. In the event of a catastrophic biological attack, however, hospitals may be overloaded. If so, seek out an alternative predesignated treatment site and get the patient there as soon as possible. These patients require treatment that may be near-impossible to provide at home, so even if the alternate site seems ill-equipped compared to a hospital, you will be better off there than going it alone. Whichever facility you ultimately use, keep in mind that if the health care pipeline is available, get the patient into the system at the onset of the illness as soon as possible, since car travel and movement can damage capillaries as the illness progresses.

In the worst-case scenario, in which public health care facilities have shut down or are unavailable, people may be on their own.

Whether in the hospital or at home, the main goal for the caretaker is to deliver appropriate drugs wherever possible, and to support the patient while avoiding infection with a highly contagious virus himself or herself.

The VHF patient will suffer confusion as a result of the illness. Despite your doubts and fears, you must reassure the victim that he or she is being cared for, and that you are doing all you can. Judicious use of pain-relieving or sedative medications may help, but avoid aspirin or any other medication that thins the blood, since this may render the symptoms—characterized by bleeding through damage to the capillary system—far worse.

VHF patients are often slightly dehydrated from heat, fever, anorexia, vomiting, and diarrhea, in any combination. There is obvious loss of blood, as well as internal blood loss you cannot even see. Severe loss of blood may lead to shock, and therefore, care will need to include infusion of fluid as well as products that enhance the ability of the blood to clot. But delivering the treatment is tricky. Despite the fact that VHF patients are losing fluid, they often respond poorly to fluid infusions and can develop pulmonary edema as a result. To avoid this outcome, rehydration should be done only with what professionals refer to as colloid or crystalloid solutions. Ringer's lactate solution is one example. Hetastarch is another. If this does not work, the U.S. Army suggests that pharmacological doses of corticosteroids (e.g., methylprednisolone 30 mg/kg) may provide another possible but untested therapy for treating shock caused by blood loss.

Dr. Rega, meanwhile, notes that hantavirus, in particular, can lead to renal failure and could require dialysis. Hantavirus can also induce symptoms similar to those of "acute respiratory distress syndrome," a condition that requires aggressive pulmonary management, including supplemental oxygen, intubation, and mechanical ventilation.

With the exception of dengue and classic hantavirus, patients with VHF syndrome generally have significant quantities of virus in their blood, and perhaps in other secretions as well. This is why secondary infections among contacts and medical caretakers are common. Thus, the caretaker must exercise extreme caution while making the victim as comfortable as possible.

Patients should be isolated, in a room of their own, and should have separate bathroom facilities. Children should be kept from adults with disease. Caretakers must use cap, gown, gloves, and mask, preferably one with a HEPA filter. In the aftermath of any attack with VHF, caretakers will surely be considered heroes for putting themselves in "the line of fire." Nonetheless, they must balance their heroism with stringent rules of self-protection, lest they not only get sick themselves but also pass the disease on.

The best lessons concerning care and treatment of the VHFs outside the modern hospital setting may come from Africa, where most of the experience has been. These lessons have been summarized by the World Health Organization in its extensive manual entitled *Infection Control for Viral Haemorrhagic Fevers in the African Health Care Setting*. If you would like to see the entire manual, simply follow the Internet link referenced in the resource guide at the end of this book. It is impossible, in this volume, to repeat everything described in that ultimate source. Suffice it to say, however, that the motto, "caretaker, protect thyself" must be your mantra and theme. If you are caring for a loved one with one of the viral hemorrhagic fevers, remember that you may become the next victim if you do not guard against contact with the patient's respiratory drops, bodily fluids, or even sweat. If you are a caregiver, says Dr. Rega, you must check yourself for fever twice daily. In Africa, those who come in contact with Ebola victims are monitored for 21 days.

Even though most care is supportive, antiviral medication has been shown to work for some of the VHFs. The antiviral drug ribavirin has been shown to be effective for treating Lassa virus, the South American hemorrhagic fever viruses including Junin virus, and hantavirus as well as Bolivian, Crimean-Congo, and Rift Valley hemorrhagic fevers. Antiviral agents have not been shown to be effective in treating infections caused by Ebola or Marburg virus or the flaviviruses, including yellow fever and dengue. The earlier in the course of the illness the medication can be delivered, the more likely it is to help. It is most useful within 7 days of onset. In the case of hantavirus, treatment should begin within 4 days.

The recommended regimen for an infected individual is:

- Ribavirin, 30 mg/kg intravenously (IV) as a loading dose.
- Then 16 mg/kg IV every 6 hours for 4 days.
- Then 8 mg/kg IV every 8 hours for 6 days (total treatment time of 10 days).

Ribavirin may be useful for close contacts of a patient with Lassa fever (500 mg orally every 6 hours for 7 days), according to the CDC guideline "Management of Patients with Suspected Viral Hemorrhagic Fever." No therapy for postexposure prophylaxis is available for Marburg or Ebola viruses.

Important note: Ribavirin may be harmful to the fetus, but in instances where the mother has been diagnosed with a definite case of viral hemorrhagic fever, it is the recommended treatment, nonetheless. Finally, because Ribavirin does not pass the blood-brain barrier, it may be ineffective against neurological symptoms.

According to the U.S. Army, it is worth noting that there have been near-miraculous anecdotal reports of recovery based on treatment with "passive immunization"—treatment with plasma taken from individuals who have contracted and survived the disease. "This approach has often been taken in desperation, owing to the limited availability of effective antiviral drugs," says the Army's Peter Jahrling, adding that "anecdotal case reports describing miraculous successes are frequently tempered by more systematic studies, where efficacy is less obvious." For all VHF viruses, the benefit of this treatment depends upon the concentration of antibodies in the plasma used. Some, but not all, VHFs induce the antibodies in the blood of those they infect.

Clearly, it would be impossible for an individual at home to whip up this plasma outside of the health care pipeline. But those with access to medical professionals and hospitals might be able, in the absense of ribavirin, to fall back on passive immunity, as detailed below:

- Argentine hemorrhagic fever responds to therapy with two or more units of convalescent plasma containing adequate amounts of neutralizing antibody provided that treatment is initiated within 8 days of the time symptoms start.
- Antibody therapy is beneficial in the treatment of Bolivian hemorrhagic fever.
- This approach will not work with hantavirus, since these patients

arc already developing immune responses of their own by the time they are recognized; it will not be possible for antibody-loaded plasma to circumvent a natural process that has already begun.

The only established and licensed virus-specific vaccine available against any of the hemorrhagic fever viruses is the yellow fever vaccine, which is mandatory for travelers to areas of Africa and South America where the virus is epidemic. Other vaccines exist, but they are experimental. Investigational vaccines have shown some utility against Argentine hemorrhagic fever, Junin, Bolivian hemorrhagic fever, Rift Valley fever, Hantaan virus, and dengue.

Though yellow fever vaccine has been approved and is available to the public, recent reports warn of a shortage. The issue isn't always clear to American tourists, who freely receive the vaccine when needed. But in case of a true outbreak or epidemic, say the experts, there wouldn't be anywhere near enough to go around. The potential for trouble is highlighted in the December 22, 2001 issue of the *Lancet,* where Nicolas Nathan and a team of scientists from *Epicentre* in Paris describe events surrounding a yellow fever epidemic in Guinea.

From September 4, 2000, to January 7, 2001, 688 people came down with yellow fever in Guinea, with 225 ultimately succumbing to the disease. The best defense would have been a mass vaccination campaign, but it was limited due to insufficient international stocks—in fact, although the vaccine effort was spearheaded by the World Health Organization and UNICEF, and although the vaccine was brought in from Europe, from the Pasteur Dakar institute, and from national stocks in Niger, Nigeria, and Ghana, there still was not enough to inoculate the target population.

Luckily for Guinea, the extent of the outbreak was minor compared to other, recent epidemics. For instance, there were 100,000 cases reported in Ethiopia in 1960, 20,000 in Senegal in 1965, and 100,000 in Nigeria in 1969. Between 1986 and 1994, more than 20,000 cases were reported in successive epidemics in Nigeria. The Guinea episode revealed that we lack enough vaccine for even a small outbreak, never mind the epidemics or even pandemics that could result from a multipronged terrorist attack. At least in the aftermath of Guinea, WHO has decided to increase international stockpiles; as the bioterrorism risk is spelled out in greater detail over the next few years, the United States may decide to do the same.

What You Need to Know to Survive an Attack of Viral Hemorrhagic Fever

- Suspect VHF if symptoms include high fever and any of a number of signs of bleeding or dysfunction of the vascular system, from nosebleeds to facial flushing to jaundice.
- If you suspect VHF, avoid aspirin or any other drug that thins blood or slows clotting, since bleeding is a danger for the infected.
- Keep in mind that antiviral medication may improve the outcome.
- Intensive hospital treatment yields the best chance for survival and recovery. If your hospital is open for business, get the patient there as soon in the course of the illness as possible. The more advanced the illness, the more likely the patient is to suffer capillary damage en route to the hospital as a result of movement.
- Avoid excess movement of the patient. Careless manipulation could aggravate bruising of the skin. Any movement, even minor movement for feeding or cleaning, must be gentle.
- Avoid needle sticks, since VHF patients have trouble with blood clots and will bleed freely.
- If your hospital is overloaded, get to an alternative predesignated treatment site.
- These patients are confused and require reassurance that they are being cared for.
- In a catastrophic situation, in which true authorities may be unavailable, it will be impossible to know for sure whether a fever is caused by VHF or not, even if there has been a confirmed outbreak of VHF in your area. In that case, says the World Health Organization, patients are to be treated with 3 days of antibiotics to address a possible bacterial infection. If fever persists after 3 days, antibiotic therapy should be halted as ineffective and the VHF diagnosis can be presumed.
- If you are caring for a loved one with VHF, you are at great risk of catching infection. To avoid this outcome, minimize respiratory and other contact with the infected patient and follow protective precautions to the letter.
- VHF precautions mean that you will wear protective clothing when in the same room as the patient, and in any room where you clean or wash anything touched by the patient.
- Your protective gear will include a scrub suit, gown, apron, two

pairs of gloves (one on top of the other), mask, head cover, eye-wear like protective goggles, and rubber boots.

- If you are a caretaker, wash your hands with soap and water before and after each contact with the infected individual. Make sure you wash hands up to the forearm, and thoroughly rinse soap away with clean running water.
- All towels used for infected individuals should be discarded. Paper towels are most practical. If no paper towels are available, air dry your hands whenever possible.
- VHF organisms will grow and multiply in humidity and standing water. Therefore, if you are using cake soap, cut it into small pieces and discard after use. Liquid soap in a dispenser is a good alternative. Above all, never use soap that has been allowed to sit in a soap dish, where wet conditions will breed germs.
- Limit the family members who care for or, for that matter, have any contact with the sick person or the isolation area to the smallest number possible.
- Patients with significant vomiting, coughing, and diarrhea are more likely to infect the caregiver with their emissions.
- Unless you are instructed otherwise by medical professionals, all patients must remain in isolation until they are completely well.
- Anything emitted from a patient (mucus, sweat, phlegm, feces, urine, etc.) that has come in contact with another's skin, eyes, or mouth, should be immediately washed off or irrigated out. Ebola may even be contagious through contact with the patient's sweat.
- Caregivers must check themselves for fever twice daily.
- Subdivide areas of your house or apartment, especially if you are dealing with contagious forms of VHF. Under the best of all circumstances, you will create an isolation room for the patient; a bathroom to be used only by the patient, adjoining the isolation room; a changing room where only the caretaker can go; and a separate bathroom or sink that the caregiver can use to clean anything associated with the patient.
- If you do not have a separate bathroom for the infected individual in your home, try to set up a portable or temporary facility in the patient's room for that purpose.
- If your house has more than one door to the outside, have uninfected family members use one door and have the caretaker use a separate door.

- If your home has central air-conditioning, do not use it. You want to do all you can to make sure the virus will not be transmitted through a ventilation system.
- Report suspected cases or suspected intentional release of VHF to your local health department. The local health department is responsible for notifying the state health department, the FBI, and local law enforcement. The state health department will notify the CDC.
- Bodies of deceased victims should be cremated whenever possible.

10

The Equine Encephalitides:

Venezuelan Encephalitis (VEE), Western Encephalitis (WEE), and Eastern Encephalitis (EEE)

Delivery: Inhalation of aerosol is most likely; intentional release of infected mosquitoes has also been mentioned as a threat.

Symptoms: Flulike illness and range of neurological effects. Earliest symptoms include headache, photophobia, and muscle pain. As the diseases progress, patients may experience excess salivation, sore throat, diarrhea, nausea, and vomiting as well as confusion, lethargy, cranial nerve palsies, seizures, and impaired respiratory regulation. Meningitis and coma can be an end result. A hallmark of these diseases, especially in a weaponized version, is encephalitis (inflammation of the brain), a situation that can cause permanent neurological damage, especially in children. Chance of survival depends upon the specific type of encephalitis. In Venezuelan equine encephalitis (VEE), only 1% of adults succumb to the disease, although 20% of children who develop encephalitis from this infection will die. With western equine encephalitis (WEE), 10% of victims succumb. The most severe of these weapons is eastern equine encephalitis (EEE), which kills 50–70% of victims, with survivors often suffering permanent neurological deficit. For all three diseases, children and the elderly are the most severely affected.

Timeline: From exposure to appearance of symptoms, 1–6 days for EEE, 5–10 days for WEE, and 5–15 days for VEE.

Can be mistaken for: Flu, brucellosis, botulism, plague, salmonel-

losis, Lyme disease, and Q fever. Also, dengue, malaria, meningitis, and yellow fever.
Treatment: The only proven care is supportive. The antiviral drug ribavirin as well as alpha-interferon may be effective based on studies with animals, but actual treatment protocols are unknown. Experimental vaccines may be considered for prophylaxis, but only if the organism released is judged to be significantly lethal.

The Equine Encephalitides in Nature

It wasn't until the 1930s that researchers studying moribund horses isolated the cause of severe equine encephalitis in three distinct but related viruses: western equine encephalitis (WEE) virus in California, eastern equine encephalitis (EEE) virus in Virginia and New Jersey, and Venezuelan equine encephalitis (VEE) virus in the Guajira peninsula of Venezuela. By 1938 scientists realized this triad of microbes caused encephalitis in humans, too. Humans as well as horses, donkeys, mules, and burros contracted the disease by mosquito bite, but humans also became infected through aerosolization of the microbe in the lab. So virulent was the aerosol version that when a few vials of VEE were dropped in a stairwell of the Ivanovskii Institute in Moscow in 1959, 20 workers took ill in a day and a half.

The equine encephalitides have caused plenty of havoc in the natural world. Between 1969 and 1971, a virulent VEE strain emerged in Guatemala, moved through Mexico, and entered Texas, all the while infecting both equine species and humans. There were 8,000–10,000 equine deaths, tens of thousands of equine cases, and 17,000 human cases in Mexico alone. When more than 10,000 horses died in Texas, however, the U.S. government got involved.

Before the United States was done, it had developed a vaccine, vaccinated 95% of all horses and donkeys (some 3.2 million animals), established equine quarantines, and controlled mosquito populations through insecticide use in the Rio Grande Valley and along the Gulf Coast. While the United States was now protected from this scourge, a second VEE outbreak in 1995 in Venezuela and Colombia involved over 75,000 human cases and over 20 deaths.

The Equine Encephalitides as Weapons of Biological Terror

Owing to their natural attributes, the equine encephalitides have long been considered ideal for the arsenal of biological war. One clear advantage derives from their ability to thrive in so many diverse hosts in nature, from horses to mosquitoes to humans. This broad-based ability to survive in so many environments also means these microbes can survive under a diversity of circumstances in the lab. According to the U.S. Army, a billion infectious units per milliliter are not unusual; what's more, it may require no more than 10–100 such organisms to provoke disease. Easy to grow and study in the test tube, these encephalitides have served as model organisms to help scientists understand viral pathogenesis in general. In the process, researchers came to know these species, especially VEE, particularly well, making it all the more possible to culture them anywhere and hone and improve them to specific ends.

The U.S. Army has listed the strategic advantages of VEE, WEE, and EEE in its textbook *Medical Aspects of Chemical and Biological Warfare:*

- These viruses can be produced in large amounts in inexpensive and unsophisticated systems.
- They are relatively stable and highly infectious for humans as aerosols.
- Available strains produce either incapacitating or lethal infections.
- The existence of multiple versions of VEE and EEE viruses, as well as the inherent difficulties of inducing efficient immunity, confounds defensive vaccine development.

The equine encephalatides remain as "highly credible threats today, and intentional release as a small-particle aerosol, from a single airplane, could be expected to infect a high percentage of individuals within an area of at least 10,000 km," the textbook states. Susceptibility is high—90–100% of those who inhale the "loading dose" are infected. And nearly 100% of those infected develop overt illnesses. "As a further complication, these viruses are readily amenable to genetic manipulation by modern recombinant deoxyribonucleic acid (DNA) technology. This capability is being used to develop safer and more effective vaccines, but in theory could also be used to increase the weaponization potential of these viruses."

It's well known, these days, that the United States itself grew VEE in chicken eggs, then aerosolized and stockpiled it as part of its biological warfare program at Fort Detrick until the effort was disbanded in 1969. Today the United States says its supply of weaponized VEE has been destroyed.

Of less comfort is the report of Ken Alibek, once in charge of the Soviet biological warfare program. He recalls efforts to create "chimeras" in which genes from VEE were inserted into the body of a smallpoxlike virus. In the 1980s, said Alibek, the Soviets used the ectromelia virus as a model for smallpox. "A chimera strain of ectromelia and VEE was created for initial testing. The tests indicated that this chimera strain simultaneously caused symptoms of both ectromelia and VEE in subject animals." The Soviets later inserted VEE into vaccinia (cowpox) virus, considered a strong model for smallpox because the two are so much alike. While no one knows the status of this work, Alibek has recently said he believes the Russians may be "continuing to carry out the research and concealment plans that were in place prior to my departure for the United States in 1992."

Signs and Symptoms

Given extensive laboratory experience and known efforts at weaponization, VEE remains the most likely of the equine encephalitides to be used as a weapon of biological war. But in terms of clinical presentation, it makes little difference, for presentation of all three viruses will be essentially the same. Symptoms will start suddenly with a severe, incapacitating illness marked by spiking high fever, exhaustion, chills, muscle pain, and extreme sensitivity to light. Nausea, vomiting, cough, sore throat, and diarrhea may follow. Patients would be incapacitated by malaise and fatigue for 1–2 weeks before full recovery. In the end, the distinction will be not so much between the three viruses as between natural infection and infection manufactured for war. In natural disease, most EEE and WEE patients but only a small percentage of VEE patients present with encephalitis; with weaponized VEE, on the other hand, encephalitic presentation is expected to be high.

Indeed, during natural VEE epidemics just 4% of infected children and less than 1% of adults will develop signs of severe central nervous system infection (35% fatality for children and 10% for adults in this severe form of the disease). But the experts say that experimental aerosol challenges of a biological attack will probably have a far higher incidence of central nervous system disease and the associated death rate that results.

How can you recognize the presence of central nervous system disease? Mild CNS symptoms include lethargy, somnolence, and mild confusion. Severe CNS involvement might result in seizures, paralysis, or coma. During pregnancy, weaponized VEE could result in miscarriage, damage to the placenta, and encephalitis or even severe neuroanatomical defects in the unborn child.

As with many other weapons of biological war, an outbreak of EEE, WEE, or VEE would at first be difficult to distinguish from influenza. Physicians might not suspect the encephalitides until a proportion of the "flu" patients came down with neurological symptoms, including seizures and coma.

How Medical Professionals Diagnose the Equine Encephalitides

Physicians will first suspect these diseases based on symptoms and presumed risk of infection. But the diagnosis will ultimately be confirmed in the lab by isolating the virus or through blood tests that detect antibodies or use polymerase chain reaction to analyze DNA. The difficulty of these kinds of tests during national emergency, when the health delivery system is already stressed, is the need for labs with enough security to protect technicians from themselves contracting the disease. Other signs, including low white blood cell count and elevated protein and pressure in cerebral spinal fluid, can be at least suggestive that an equine encephalitide is at the root of the disease.

Care and Treatment

Unlike the viral hemorrhagic fevers, researchers have found no evidence of human-to-human transmission for the equine encephalitides. Therefore, patient isolation and quarantine is not required. To prevent spread of the disease, however, patients must be treated in screened rooms to prevent the entry of mosquitoes, which may pick up infection by biting the patient and then spread it to others. The Army also recommends use of a residual insecticide in the patient's room for at least 5 days after symptoms begin or until fever subsides.

Because there is no proven drug therapy, the mainstay of treatment remains supportive care. Patients with uncomplicated infection should be treated with analgesics to relieve headache and muscle pain, according to the Army's *Medical Management of Biological Casualties Handbook*. Patients who develop encephalitis may require anticonvulsants and electrolytes to maintain fluid and electrolyte balance. Because the encephalitides can depress the immune system, these patients must be tested and treated for secondary bacterial infections.

There is also some preliminary evidence in animals that ribavirin, alpha-interferon, and the interferon-inducer poly-ICLC may be of therapeutic value. But researchers lack any clinical data on which to base the efficacy of these drugs in humans. Indeed, the information is so new and preliminary that treatment guidelines are unavailable. Should terrorists strike with VEE, WEE, or EEE, however, specific dosing schedules may evolve on the fly, as they have with the recent anthrax outbreak, where the book on treatment has been rewritten since September 11, 2001.

The best advice available regarding these medications is to call the CDC at 1-770-488-7100 or the Army at 1-888-872-7443 to see what they recommend at the time. As to management of these medications, if the public health pipeline has not responded in terms of specific treatment protocols or sufficient stockpile, you should make sure you reach a tertiary care center like a teaching or university hospital as soon as possible. If you do not have a tertiary care center nearby, simply get to the nearest hospital.

As to vaccines, these are available in experimental versions only, including a live attenuated vaccine for VEE (TC-83) and inactivated vaccines for VEE, EEE, and WEE. These vaccines are useful for at-risk individuals, such as those regularly exposed to these pathogens in the laboratory. But they do not always work and are associated with significant side effects. Moreover, it is questionable how effective these vaccines would be in the face of a biological attack. After all, as with all vaccines, the degree of protection depends upon the magnitude of the challenge dose; vaccine-induced protection could be overwhelmed by extremely high doses of the pathogen. New vaccines are being researched, but are unavailable at this time.

What You Need to Know to Survive an Attack of VEE, EEE, or WEE

- As part of your advance preparation, determine the location of the closest tertiary care hospital in your area. Also note the location of hospitals with the most extensive emergency departments and the greatest number of board certified emergency physicians. (Board certification signifies specific competence in the field of emergency medicine.) These should be your destinations of choice in the event you think you have been infected with one of the equine encephalitides.
- If you or a family member present with neurological symptoms, get to a tertiary care center to be checked out as soon as possible.
- Keep in mind that not every individual with neurological symptoms will have been infected with one of the equine encephalitides, even if they are in the vicinity of an attack. These neurological symptoms could also be a sign of stroke, hypoxia (deficiency of oxygen reaching the tissues of the body), botulism, or any number of other health problems.
- Patients must be treated in screened rooms to prevent the entry of mosquitoes, which may pick up infection by biting the patient and then spread it to others.
- Patients with uncomplicated infection should be treated with analgesics to relieve headache and muscle pain.
- Patients who develop encephalitis may require anticonvulsants and electrolytes to maintain fluid and electrolyte balance.
- Animal research indicates that ribavirin, alpha-interferon, and the interferon-inducer poly-ICLC may be of therapeutic value, although there are no treatment guidelines for humans.
- There is no evidence of human-to-human transmission. Nonetheless, it's helpful to keep in mind that VEE, EEE, and WEE are all killed with heat and ordinary household disinfectants.
- Report suspected cases or suspected intentional release of an equine encephalitide to your local health department. The local health department is responsible for notifying the state health department, the FBI, and local law enforcement. The state health department will notify the CDC.

THE TOXINS

Toxins are poisonous by-products of living organisms, including microbes, plants, and animals. They are very stable and produce severe illness when ingested, inhaled, or introduced into the body by any other means. Their effects on the human body range from minor illness to death. They differ from chemical agents because they are not man-made, are not explosive, and do not emit vapors. Many toxins also pack more bang for the buck than chemical agents, with the most toxic of the toxins significantly more damaging than the most lethal chemical agent. They differ from other biological weapons because they cannot replicate and thus cannot be passed from one person to the next.

11

Botulism

Delivery: Aerosol or sabotage of food supply.

Symptoms: The botulism victim at first presents as awake and alert and without fever, but with what physicians call "descending symmetrical paralysis." This means that paralysis starts at the top of the head and moves down. First the individual will experience drooping eyelids, with paralysis later affecting the throat, the arms and hands, and finally the legs. As paralysis advances, symptoms may include drooping eyelids, altered voice, disturbance of speech and language, and difficulty swallowing. Also look for double vision, extreme aversion to light, and dry mouth. If the toxin is food-borne, delayed symptoms will include nausea, vomiting, diarrhea, and cramping. The end stage involves paralysis, respiratory failure, and death. Botulism does not cause fever, so if you have a fever, look for another cause.

Timeline: From exposure to appearance of symptoms, the range is variable, from a few hours to 5 days. With ingestion, usually 24–36 hours, and if toxin is inhaled. Death within 3 days, but if not fatal symptoms may last months. Full recovery up to a year.

Can be mistaken for: Myasthenia gravis, Guillain-Barré syndrome, Eaton-Lambert syndrome, tick paralysis, stroke, organophosphate poisoning, atropine poisoning, polio, and mushroom poisoning.

Treatment: A range of antitoxins.

Botulism in Nature

Botulinum toxins are a group of seven toxins produced by an anaerobic bacterium called *Clostridium (C.) botulinum*. Ubiquitous in nature, the bacterial spores germinate in soil, animals, and fish to give rise to vegetative bacteria that produce toxins during incubation. The organisms can be recovered from honey and other agricultural products. The highest-risk foods are improperly canned foods and dried meat or fish.

Naturally occurring botulism is the disease that results from the absorption of botulinum toxin into the circulation from a mucosal surface (gut, lung) or a wound. It does not penetrate intact skin. The toxin irreversibly binds to synapses, the connectors that enable one neuron to communicate with another. As a result, they prevent release of the neurotransmitter acetylcholine from motor neurons, leading to muscle paralysis and, in severe cases, the need for mechanical respiration.

Botulinum toxin can be grouped into seven categories, designated A through G depending upon the strain of *Clostridia botulinum* used. The categories are especially important because you can only neutralize an A toxin with anti-A toxin, a B toxin with anti-B toxin, and so on.

Natural cases of botulism are rare. They most frequently result from food contamination, although they may derive from wounds and lack of gastrointestinal microflora as well. A thumbnail summary follows:

Food-borne Botulism   Food-borne botulism is due to ingestion of food contaminated with botulinum toxins. Inadequately heating vegetables and fruits during canning, then inadequate heating before serving is the primary mode of transmission in the United States. In some foreign countries, smoked sausage, salmon, and fermented salmon eggs are the source of intoxication. In Asian countries, seafood is the primary source of intoxication, which typically results from food contamination. Many types of food have been associated with outbreaks in the past, with the common factor being that implicated food items were not heated or were incompletely heated. Heat of 185°F or more inactivates the toxin. (The largest botulism outbreak in the United States in the past century occurred in 1977, when 59 people became ill from poorly preserved jalapeño peppers. No cases of waterborne botulism have ever been reported. This is likely due to the large amount of toxin needed, and the fact that the toxin is easily neutralized by common water treatment techniques.)

Infantile Botulism   Germination of spores leading to colonization and toxin production may occur in the infantile gastrointestinal (GI) tract owing to anatomic, physiologic, and microbiologic factors present during the first year of life. *Clostridium botulinum* spores survive transit through the stomach and can then germinate and colonize the intestinal tract in the absence of well-established GI tract microflora. Parents are advised not to feed infants honey, molasses, and other foods potentially high in *C. botulinum* spore content. This form of botulism is a rare disease of adults but may occur in cases of underlying anatomic or physiologic abnormalities of the GI tract, or alteration of the normal GI tract flora (such as after antibiotic exposure).

Wound Botulism   Wound botulism is due to the germination of *C. botulinum* spores and subsequent production of toxin in traumatic wounds. The spores may be introduced by organisms entering during wounding, by drug abusers who infect injection sites, and by cocaine abusers inhaling the spores into nasal ulcers and sinuses.

Botulism can also present as a less serious illness, limited to cranial nerve palsies and mild gastrointestinal symptoms.

Botulism as a Weapon of Biological Terror

According to the Working Group on Civilian Biodefense and the *Journal of the American Medical Association*, "botulinum toxin poses a major bioweapon threat because of its extreme potency and lethality; its ease of production, transport, and misuse; and the need for prolonged intensive care among affected persons. An outbreak of botulism constitutes a medical emergency that requires prompt provision of botulinum antitoxin and, often, mechanical ventilation, and it constitutes a public health emergency that requires immediate intervention to prevent additional cases."

As the most poisonous substance known, crystalline botulinum toxin in the amount of a single gram, evenly dispersed and inhaled, would kill more than a million people, according to the Working Group. Those who survived would require prolonged intensive care. To give you an idea of its potency, botulism is 275 times more toxic than cyanide, and 100,000 times more toxic than sarin nerve gas, used by the Aum Shinrikyo group in Japan to kill 12 people in the Tokyo subway system in 1995.

What's more, botulism has already been weaponized, and sits ready for deployment around the world. In fact, terrorists have already attempted to use botulinum toxin as a bioweapon, according to the *JAMA* Working Group. Aerosols were dispersed at multiple sites in downtown Tokyo, Japan, and at U.S. military installations in Japan on at least three occasions between 1990 and 1995 by Aum Shinrikyo. "These attacks failed, apparently because of faulty microbiological technique, deficient aerosol-generating equipment, or internal sabotage," the *Journal* says, adding that "the perpetrators obtained their *C. botulinum* from soil that they had collected in northern Japan."

But this toxin is not new to the Japanese. The head of the Japanese biological warfare group admitted to feeding cultures of *C. botulinum* to prisoners with lethal effect during that country's occupation of Manchuria, which began in the 1930s. The U.S. biological weapons program, meanwhile, first produced botulinum toxin during World War II. In fact, the United States was so concerned that Germany had weaponized botulinum toxin during the war that it made more than a million doses of vaccine for Allied troops preparing to invade Normandy on D-Day. Although the United States is said to have destroyed its botulinum stockpiles along with the rest of its germ arsenal in 1969, Thomas Inglesby, M.D., a researcher with the Center for Civilian Biodefense Studies and assistant professor of infectious diseases at Johns Hopkins School of Medicine, notes that several nations, including Russia and Iraq, signatories to the Biological Weapons Convention, have developed and stockpiled botulinum toxin weapons that are ready for use.

The Working Group provided details in *JAMA*: Botulinum toxin was one of several agents tested at the Soviet site Aralsk-7 on Vozrozhdeniye Island in the Aral Sea, they note, pointing as well to the testimony of Ken Alibek, the former senior scientist of the Russian civilian bioweapons program. Alibek reported that the Soviets had attempted splicing the botulinum toxin gene from *C. botulinum* into other bacteria, hoping to engineer a contagious form of the illness. Their efforts are even more worrisome because thousands of the Soviet biowarfare scientists were left without work following the demise of the USSR, and some have reportedly been recruited by other countries with aspirations of stockpiling weapons of biological war.

There is little doubt that four of them—Iran, Iraq, North Korea, and Syria, all labeled state sponsors of terrorism by the U.S. State Department—have developed, or are in the process of developing, weaponized botulism. Iraq admitted that much to the United Nations inspection team in 1991, in the aftermath of the Persian Gulf War. Indeed, Iraq conceded having produced 19,000 liters of concentrated botulinum toxin, including 10,000 liters loaded into military weapons and ready to fly.

"These 19,000 liters of concentrated toxin are not fully accounted for," according to the *JAMA* Working Group, "and constitute approximately 3 times the amount needed to kill the entire current human population by inhalation." The Group also reports that in 1990, Iraq deployed specially designed missiles with a 600-km range; 13 of these were filled with botulinum toxin, 10 with aflatoxin, and 2 with anthrax spores. "Iraq also deployed special 400-lb (180-kg) bombs for immediate use; 100 bombs contained botulinum toxin, 50 contained anthrax spores, and 7 contained aflatoxin," says *JAMA*. "It is noteworthy that Iraq chose to weaponize more botulinum toxin than any other of its known biological agents."

Based on wide-ranging analysis, *JAMA* concludes that botulinum toxin would be more effective against civilian populations than against military troops. One estimate, for instance, contends that a release of botulinum aerosol would kill or incapacitate 10% of those within 0.5 kilometers downwind—not enough to stop an army, but certainly sufficient to create public mayhem and halt a society in its tracks. Add this to the notion that smaller, multiple efforts could introduce the toxin into the food supply around the United States, and you have a recipe for disaster in the public realm.

Signs and Symptoms

The botulism victim at first presents as awake and alert and without fever, but with what physicians call "descending symmetrical paralysis." This means that paralysis starts from the top of the head, manifesting in drooping eyelids, and moving down to affect the throat, the arms and hands, and finally the legs. Paralysis from botulism poisoning differs essentially from paralysis from stroke. In stroke, where one side or just part of the brain is affected, observers will see selective paralysis that affects just one part or one side of the body. The paralysis is decidedly asymmetrical. With botulism, on the other hand, paralysis is equally distributed on the left and right sides of the body as it travels from head to toe. As paralysis advances, symptoms may include ptosis (drooping eyelids), dysphonia (altered voice), dysarthria (disturbance of speech and language), and dysphagia (difficulty swallowing). Also look for double vision, photophobia (extreme aversion to light), and dry mouth. If the toxin is food-borne, delayed symptoms will include nausea, vomiting, diarrhea, and cramping. Botulism kills almost solely by paralyzing the muscles involved with breathing. The end stage involves paralysis, respiratory failure, and death. Botulism does not cause fever, so if you have a fever, look for another cause.

Exposed individuals may initially present with difficulty swallowing, progressive weakness, nausea, vomiting, abdominal cramps, and difficulty breathing, sometimes followed by periods of apnea or a total cessation of breathing. Blurred vision and other neurological symptoms are common as well. Symptoms are similar for all toxin types, but the severity of illness can vary widely, in part depending on the amount of toxin absorbed. Recovery from paralysis can take from weeks to months and requires the growth of new motor nerve endings. The infected may need to spend months on a respirator if they hope to survive.

How Medical Professionals Diagnose Botulism

A deliberate aerosol or food-borne release of botulinum toxin could be detected by several features: a large number of acute cases presenting all at once; cases involving an uncommon toxin type (C, D, F, G, or non-aquatic-food-associated E); patients from the same geographic area but without a common dietary exposure; and multiple simultaneous outbreaks without a common source.

Laboratory diagnosis and testing are available at the CDC and some local and state facilities. Clinical and food specimens can be tested directly for botulinum toxin or can be cultured for *C. botulinum* with subsequent toxin testing of isolates from those cultures. In addition, labs can test the infected by analyzing serum, stool, vomit, expired gases, or material from wounds. Toxin testing is performed using the "mouse bioassay," which involves injecting mice with material from clinical specimens or food and using type-specific antitoxin to demonstrate protection.

Other tests may be useful in distinguishing botulism from other illnesses. The electromyelogram may show several characteristic features, including an incremental response to repetitive nerve stimulation, normal sensory function, normal nerve-conduction velocity, and a characteristic pattern of small-amplitude motor potentials. Physicians may also rule out other illnesses through a spinal tap; in the botulism patient, spinal tap will be normal.

Despite all the options, botulism must remain a clinical diagnosis based on symptoms because laboratory testing is time consuming, so much so that waiting for the results would be a death sentence to anyone actually infected. If there is a high index of suspicion, including a known bioterrorist attack, patients with symptoms should be treated first and have their diagnosis confirmed later.

Care and Treatment

Botulism is not contagious, and caretakers for these extremely sick individuals are not themselves at risk for catching the disease.

In the event there is clinical suspicion that you are a victim of botulinum toxin, treatment with antitoxin must begin at once. In the United States, licensed botulinum equine antitoxin is available from the CDC via state and local health departments. Your health department can be contacted via the phone numbers at the back of this book.

The licensed trivalent antitoxin contains neutralizing antibodies against botulinum toxin types A, B, and E, the most common causes of human botulism. If another toxin type were intentionally disseminated, patients could potentially be treated with heptavalent antitoxin, an experimental drug held by the U.S. Army that covers types A through G. (Keep in mind that the time required for toxin typing would decrease the utility of this version.)

Experts say that existing technologies could produce large reserves of human antibody against the botulinum toxin. Administration of such a therapy could provide immunity of up to a month or greater and eliminate the need for rationing. But at the moment, that effort is woefully late in getting off the ground.

For this reason, if you suspect you have been exposed to botulism, you must make sure you are first on line to receive antitoxin from the health delivery establishment. In the event of a true and widespread attack, antitoxin might be available on a first come, first served basis, and you'll want to make sure you are treated before supplies run out.

Is there any way an individual can stock a small amount of botulism antitoxin at home? Absolutely not. The CDC maintains the supply.

While antitoxin delivered upon exposure would prevent symptoms, experts say there probably is not enough antitoxin around at this juncture to take that tack. Instead, it is likely, in any catastrophic situation, that antitoxin will not be used for prophylaxis but will be saved for those who are actually sick. This may not be as alarming as it sounds, as long as your hospital has enough antitoxin on hand to treat the sick: only 8% of those treated after onset of symptoms die.

Dosing for antitoxins has changed over time, and continues to change. Current recommendations follow, but please note these are considered an ever-changing "work in progress" by clinicians:

- For the licensed trivalent antitoxin (A, B, and E) the dose is a single 10-cc vial per patient, diluted 1:10 in 0.9% saline solution and adminstered by slow IV infusion. One vial provides antitoxin for all three types.
- For the Army's experimental, heptavalent antitoxin (to treat A–G) the dose is also a 10-cc vial delivered by IV.

Both antidotes provide far more antitoxin than is required in the instance of food poisoning, but it's not clear that this will be the case for inhalational botulism delivered by terrorists. In this instance, the patient must be retested for the presence of toxin after treatment.

For both antitoxins, patients should be screened for hypersensitivity with a small challenge dose before receiving a full dose. Patients responding to the challenge with a substantial reaction may be desensitized over 3 to 4 hours before additional antitoxin is given. During the infusion of antitoxin, diphenhydramine and epinephrine should be on hand for rapid administration in case of adverse reaction.

For prophylaxis, treat with pentavalent toxoid (A–E) experimental. This induces immunity over several months. Therefore, cases that are asymptomatic but exposed should be under close medical observation.

Do keep in mind that antitoxin works only with botulinum that has not yet bound to cells. Once the botulism toxin binds to cells, it will persist in damage. Antitoxin will not work; only supportive therapy, especially respiratory support and ventilation, will see the patient through.

Supportive care for patients with botulism may include mechanical ventilators in the intensive care unit, intravenous nutrition, and treatment of secondary bacterial infections with antibiotics. If you are being cared for by physicians in the organized health care pipeline in a coordinated effort with the CDC and your state health department, you have an excellent chance of surviving and recovering your health, even if you are almost totally paralyzed from the attack.

However, in the event of a large outbreak of botulism due to terrorist activity, the need for antitoxin, mechanical ventilators, critical care beds, and skilled personnel might quickly exceed local capacity and persist for weeks or months. Should that happen, you and your family would be on your own. Even in this situation, however, you can increase chances of survival with a few vital tips.

One issue is the use of antibiotics. These have no role in treating botulism itself. However, victims often come down with secondary bacterial infections requiring antibiotic treatment. Should this be the case, remember to avoid aminoglycoside antibiotics (e.g., streptomycin and gentamicin) and clindamycin; these can exacerbate the primary symptom of botulism, neuromuscular blockade.

Some experts also suggest that special positioning can circumvent the need for mechanical ventilation in some patients. The position requires a mattress tilted at 20 degrees, with the head part of the mattress higher than the foot. The mattress should be flat and rigid. A tightly rolled cloth should be placed under the neck to support the cervical vertebrae. Bumpers or an upright board should be placed at the feet to prevent the patient from sliding downward. Because the patient may have little or no muscular stability, you must strap the patient to the apparatus so that he doesn't crumple down to the bottom. (For toddlers and small children, you can use a crib.)

HOW TO RECOGNIZE RESPIRATORY DISTRESS

For adults and adolescents:

1. A respiratory rate of less than 10 breaths per minute. Fast breathing shows that the patient is trying to compensate and still has strength, but a very slow rate is especially troubling.
2. Perspiration.
3. Abnormal breathing, characterized by sounds like wheezing or gurgling.
4. The inability to complete sentences without taking multiple breaths.

(continued)

5. Abnormal blue or gray skin around the mouth and nailbeds.
6. Cloudiness of thinking, inability to concentrate.
7. Restlessness.
8. Use of accessory muscles in neck and abdomen to help with the mechanics of breathing.
9. A fast heartbeat that becomes increasingly slower, finally decreasing to less than 50 beats per minute.

For infants and small children:

1. Breathing noises such as wheezing or grunting.
2. Retractions of muscles in the neck, abdomen, and between ribs.
3. Poor feeding.
4. Weak cry.
5. Pale gray or blue color around mouth, fingers and toes.
6. Nasal flaring (nostrils widen with each breath).
7. Decreased activity.
8. Perspiration.
9. Poor eye contact.

If you are caring for a patient at home, it may be impossible to obtain the kind of ventilation equipment required for long-term recuperation, especially if health care systems have been compromised in a catastrophe. Your best bet is to provide temporary help until the cavalry arrives.

If a botulism patient has stopped breathing, he can be kept going with mouth-to-mouth breathing and cardiopulmonary rescuscitation until emergency medical technicians arrive. If hospitals are unavailable, you may request that EMTs intubate the patient and outfit with an ambu-bag, a temporary breath pump, of sorts, to be used as long as possible until hospitalization is possible.

Caretakers must do all they possibly can to have these patients hospitalized; without hospitalization to treat breathing problems, a high percentage of botulism patients experiencing respiratory failure will die.

On the off chance you can arrange for ventilation through alternate means, as a last-ditch effort you may contact the knowledgeable organizations listed at the end of the resource guide.

What You Need to Know to Survive an Attack of Botulism

- If you think you may have symptoms of botulism, seek hospital treatment as soon as possible. Sixty percent of those with symptoms will die without antitoxin and/or ventilatory support.
- If you have been victim of an overt attack of botulinum toxin, immediately undress and shower with soap and shampoo.
- Use household bleach for gross or visible contamination on the body.
- Put on gloves and clean any parts of the environment that have been contaminated with household bleach.
- If you fear botulism in food, heat food to 185°F for 5 minutes.
- Under conditions of terrorist attack, hospital beds, antitoxin, and ventilators may be in short supply, and you may be in the position of caring for your family without the needed medical support.
- To aid breathing, position patients on a flat, rigid mattress at a 20-degree angle from the floor, with the head higher than the feet. Place a tightly rolled cloth under the neck to support the cervical vertebrae. Place bumpers or an upright board at the foot of the bed to prevent the patient from sliding downward.
- Victims often come down with secondary bacterial infections requiring antibiotic treatment. Should this be the case, remember to avoid aminoglycoside antibiotics including streptomycin and gentamicin and clindamycin; these can exacerbate the primary symptom of botulism, neuromuscular blockade.
- If you have been on long-term antibiotic treatment, you may lack protective gastrointestinal bacteria that mitigate the effects of food-borne botulism.
- Recognition of a covert release of finely aerosolized botulinum toxin would probably occur too late to prevent additional exposures. But when you anticipate an attack, you can protect yourself, at least in part, by covering your nose and mouth with clothing like an undershirt, shirt, scarf, or handkerchief.
- While mucosal surfaces can be a conduit for infection during an attack of botulism, intact skin is impermeable to botulinum toxin.
- If you are in the position of responding to a botulism threat, take standard precautions: wash hands; wear gloves, face mask, and cap and gown.

- Clean and disinfect environmental surfaces.
- Anyone who may have been exposed should be placed in isolation until they have been decontaminated.
- Depending on the weather, aerosolized toxin has been estimated to decay at between less than 1% and 4% per minute. At a decay rate of 1% per minute, substantial inactivation of toxin occurs by 2 days after aerosolization.
- To facilitate distribution of scarce antitoxin following the intentional use of botulinum toxin, asymptomatic persons who are believed to have been exposed should remain under close medical observation and, if feasible, near critical care services.
- If you suspect botulism, contact your health department, the FBI, and local law enforcement.

12

Yellow Rain (T-2 Mycotoxin)

Delivery: Aerosol or sabotage of food supply.
Symptoms: Skin pain, itching, blisters, sneezing, cough, wheezing, chest pain. Severe intoxication results in prostration, weakness, collapse, shock, and death.
Timeline: Symptoms start anywhere from seconds to a few hours after exposure of the sort likely to result from bioterrorism.
Can be mistaken for: Ricin, staphylococcal enterotoxin B, mustard agent, or any chemical agent that gives virtually immediate signs and symptoms. Also note that SEB and ricin do not cause dermatological symptoms, while T-2 does. (T2 on skin has a color to it, generally yellowish. Other toxins generally do not have a color.)
Treatment: Soap and water; superactivated charcoal, vitamin C.

T-2 Mycotoxins in Nature

Mycotoxins, the toxic products of molds, have been implicated in health problems for decades. As an enemy, the trichothecene (T-2) mycotoxins—a group of over 40 compounds produced by the genus *Fusar-*

ium, a common grain mold—can be particularly fierce. The only class of toxin that acts directly on the skin, they cause blisters in minutes to hours after exposure. But that's just for starters. The progression of symptoms encompasses a wide range of organs and includes diarrhea, weight loss, nervous disorders, cardiovascular alterations, depression of the immune system, impairment of reproductive capacity, bone marrow destruction, and ultimately death.

The T-2 toxins do their damage in large part by inhibiting protein and nucleic acid synthesis, thus causing the same kind of sickness one often sees with radiation poisoning. As these toxins work their way through the body, they inactivate enzymes; impede the function of rapidly dividing cells like those in the bone marrow, GI tract, reproductive system, and skin; and interfere with mitochondria, the cell's energy factories. After a while, the entire body breaks down.

The T-2 mycotoxins have a special place in the annals of biological war as the deadly "yellow rain" reported and then finally documented during the 1970s and 1980s in Vietnam. But in fact, these toxins have been associated with diseases throughout history. For instance, a food-related disease has been recorded in Russia from time to time, probably since the 19th century. From 1942 through 1947, more than 10% of the population in Orenburg, near Siberia, were fatally affected by overwintered millet, wheat, and barley. The syndrome was officially named alimentary toxic aleukia (ATA). Investigation finally demonstrated that T-2 toxin, a potent trichothecene mycotoxin, was the likely agent.

The "red mold disease" of wheat and barley in Japan and associated food poisoning in people has also been attributed to the T-2 family of toxins; researchers have found trichothecenes generated by the mold species *Fusarium nivale,* isolated from grains connected with the disease. In the suburbs of Tokyo, a human illness similar to that caused by red mold was described in an outbreak of a food-borne disease, this time as a result of the consumption of *Fusarium*-infected rice.

T-2 Mycotoxins as Agents of Biological War

It is their role in biological assault, especially in Southeast Asia, that has placed the T-2 toxins high on the list of human evils. In a way it only makes sense that when scientists started searching for biological weapons, the T-2s came to mind. Extremely stable in the environment, these chemicals are not inactivated by ultraviolet light. They seem impervious to heat as well. Indeed, they retain their bioactivity even when autoclaved and cannot be destroyed unless they are heated for half an hour to 1500°F—almost twice the temperature on the planet Venus. Likewise, household bleach alone does not effectively inactivate the toxins. Rather, the addition of sodium hydroxide, the toxic chemical found in lye, would need to be added to bleach and left on a surface for an hour to have an impact—not something an untrained layperson should try to do. Fortunately, it isn't necessary. Soap and water effectively removes this oily toxin from exposed skin and other surfaces.

T-2 mycotoxins' potential for use as a weapon became abundantly clear to the Russian military prior to World War II, when flour contaminated with species of *Fusarium* was unknowingly baked into bread that was ingested by civilians. Some developed a protracted lethal illness characterized by fever, chills, and bone marrow depression. The end game was generally ugly, with the development of painful ulceration, diffuse bleeding, and the arrest of cells and organs, leading to death.

During the 1970s and 1980s, when a toxic yellow rain started falling from Laos to Afghanistan, the T-2s (and the Soviets) were blamed. Mycotoxins were allegedly released from aircraft in the yellow rain incidents in Laos (1975–81), Kampuchea (now Cambodia; 1979–81), and Afghanistan (1979–81). According to historians, attacks in Laos were directed against Hmong villagers and resistance forces who opposed the Lao People's Liberation Army and the North Vietnamese. In Kampuchea, North Vietnamese troops used T-28 aircraft to deliver toxin-filled rockets and bombs to the Khmer Rouge. The chemical munitions were supplied by the Soviets. In Afghanistan, the chemical weapons were delivered by Soviet or Afghan pilots against mujahideen guerrillas. The lethality of the attacks, the Army says, is documented by a minimum of 6,310 deaths in Laos (from 226 attacks), 981 deaths in Kampuchea (from 124 attacks), and 3,042 deaths in Afghanistan (from 47 attacks). Trichothecenes appear to have been used.

"The air attacks in Laos have been described as 'yellow rain' and consisted of a shower of sticky, yellow liquid that sounded like rain as it fell from the sky," according to the Army's report. "Other accounts described a yellow cloud of dust or powder, a mist, smoke, or insect spray–like material. Liquid agent rapidly dried to a powder. In Laos, 50% to 81% of attacks involved material associated with a yellow pigment. Other attacks were associated with red, green, white, or brown smoke or vapor. More than 80% of attacks were delivered by air-to-surface rockets; the remainder, from aircraft spray tanks or bombs. Intelligence information and some of the victims' descriptions of symptoms raised the possibility that chemical warfare agents such as phosgene, sarin, soman, mustards, and a host of other chemical incapacitants with an alphabet soup of names may also have been used. These agents may have been used in mixtures or alone."

Depite such conclusions, accounts of yellow rain in Southeast Asia have been controversial, and the Soviets denied any involvement for more than 20 years. Supporting their claims, a number of scientific experts said the deadly yellow fog was caused by bee feces, not enemy attack. It has taken years of investigation to more or less settle the controversy, documenting that the yellow rain was manufactured toxin, not swarms of migrating bees. "It is important to remember," the Army report said in evaluating that evidence, "that persons caught in a shower of bee feces do not get sick and die."

But yellow rain is not just history. T-2 toxins *still* make formidable weapons of biological war. Not only are they stable and difficult to neutralize, they can be delivered as dust, droplets, aerosols, or smoke from aircraft, rockets, missiles, artillery, mines, or portable sprayers. Appropriate for industrial-scale production, the T-2s can even be manufactured with state-of-the-art fermentation processes developed for brewing antibiotics, making it fairly simple to generate them by the ton.

Signs and Symptoms

Symptoms associated with T-2 mycotoxins vary depending upon whether exposure is chronic or acute.

Chronic exposure is the means most often found in nature, with moldy grains making their way into the food supply and catching people unawares, inflicting small doses of trichothecene mycotoxins over time. Here, the symptoms, like the toxin itself, come in stages:

Stage One From seconds to several days after consumption of contaminated grains, inflammation of the gastrointestinal tract, with vomiting, diarrhea, and abdominal pain. In most cases, excessive salivation, headache, dizziness, weakness, fatigue, and tachycardia accompany this stage, and fever and sweating may also be present.

Stage Two   Lowered white blood cell count, accompanied by decline in the function of the immune system.

Stage Three   Occurs if the individual at stage two continues to consume the contaminated food, characterized by the appearance of a bright red or dark cherry-red rash on the skin of the chest and other areas of the body. In the most severe cases, ulcers and gangrene develop in the larynx, causing the inability to speak and, ultimately, death.

Stage Four   If the individual stops consuming contaminated food, however, he or she will start to heal. In stage four of the illness—the recovery stage—body temperature will fall and lesions will heal. During this period, exposed patients are susceptible to various secondary infections, including pneumonia. Convalescence is prolonged and can last for several weeks. Usually, 2 months or more are required for the blood-forming capacity of the bone marrow to return to normal.

But it is more intensive exposure and associated acute symptoms that experts say are their major concern in the face of a terrorist attack. In the event of an out-and-out attack, acute symptoms will initially vary by delivery route: dermal exposure, local inflammation and tissue damage (a first sign that you have been exposed to T-2 in the form of yellow rain is a yellowish tint to your skin): oral exposure, lesions to the upper gastrointestinal tract; ocular exposure, and corneal injury. No matter what the route of delivery, it is important to remember that T-2 has both contact effects and systemic effects. The contact effects include irritation to mucous membranes such as eyes, nose, skin, airway, and gastrointestinal tract. The systemic effects include weakness, bone marrow suppression, and loss of coordination. Clearly, systemic symptoms indicate full-fledged T-2 disease, which can occur rapidly after exposure.

In Southeast Asia during the 1970s, according to the U.S. Army textbook *Medical Aspects of Chemical and Biological Warfare,* "symptoms began within minutes after an exploding munition caused a yellow, oily, droplet mist to fall on individuals within 100 meters of the explosion site. The falling droplet rain was inhaled, swallowed, and collected on skin and clothing; contaminated the terrain and food and water supply; and caused humans and animals to become acutely ill and to die after a variable period. Massive cutaneous contact was prevalent when the sources of exposure were sprays or coarse mists that were used deliberately to contaminate humans and the environment. Although the suspected trichothecene mycotoxin attacks in Southeast Asia would have involved multiple routes of exposure," the Army adds, "we can postulate that the skin would have been the major site for deposition of an aerosol spray or coarse mist."

Based on its experience in Southeast Asia, the Army reports that no matter what the route of exposure, early symptoms include severe nausea, vomiting, burning superficial skin discomfort, lethargy, weakness, dizziness, and loss of coordination. Within minutes to hours, you can expect diarrhea—at first watery brown and later grossly bloody. During the first 3 to 12 hours, shortness of breath, coughing, sore mouth, bleeding gums, abdominal pain, and central chest pain could occur. Exposed skin can become red, tender, swollen, or painful, in any combination, and form small or large vesicles as well as black, leathery patches. There may be tearing, pain, and conjuctivitis around the eyes. Also common are anorexia and dehydration. Dying patients experience low body heat and low blood pressure, and may have a bloody ooze from the nose and mouth. Death can occur within minutes, hours, or days and is often preceded by tremors, seizures, and coma, in any combination.

"A Canadian Forces medical team interviewed Khmer Rouge casualties after a chemical/toxin attack at Tuol Chrey, Kampuchea," the Army textbook states. "Soldiers located 100 to 300 meters from the artillery impact had onset of symptoms 2 to 5 minutes after exposure; these, likewise, included tearing, burning sensations, and blurred vision that lasted from 8 to 14 days." Analysis of autopsy samples from one of the casualties identified T-2 along with other toxins in his tissues. Culture from the autopsy was later transferred to the eyes of rabbits, causing scars on the corneas that lasted for up to five months.

Inhaling yellow rain, says the Army, translated to initial symptoms of a respiratory nature—bronchial symptoms appeared first, followed by gastrointestinal problems, including vomiting, diarrhea, abdominal pain, and acute gastroenteritis with bleeding that could be related to ingestion of the toxin. Field autopsies of victims who died 24 to 48 hours after a yellow rain attack disclosed severe gastroenteritis with bleeding in the lower esophagus and stomach, suggesting that those who succumb to inhalation of T-2 poisoning may actually die of ingestion of toxins originally deposited in the respiratory tract.

How Medical Professionals Diagnose Yellow Rain

Poisoning by T-2 mycotoxin should be suspected if you have been caught up in an aerosol attack of yellow rain with droplets of variously pigmented oily fluids contaminating clothes and the environment. Confirmation of T-2 exposure requires testing of blood, tissue, and environmental samples.

According to the U.S. Army, clinical and epidemiological findings will provide clues to the diagnosis. These include dead animals of multiple species and physical evidence such as yellow, red, green, or other pigmented oily liquid. Also supportive of diagnosis in the context of these signs is rapid onset of symptoms in minutes to hours. Mustard and other chemical agents should also be considered in any diagnosis. To confirm the diagnosis, physicians can send urine or blood to a reference lab for antigen detection. Specimens may include blood, urine, lung, liver, and stomach contents. Environmental and clinical samples can be tested using a gas liquid chromatography/mass spectrometry technique.

Care and Treatment

There is no specific antidote for T-2 mycotoxins, and treatment is therefore supportive. If you have been exposed, remove and discard all the clothes you were wearing, and shower thoroughly with soap and shampoo. Soap-and-water washing, even 4–6 hours after exposure, can significantly reduce toxicity through the skin; washing within 1 hour may prevent toxicity entirely.

You should also get to a hospital or health care facility as soon as possible. Individuals exposed to a yellow rain–like attack should be treated with standardized clinical toxicology and emergency medicine practices for ingestion of toxic compounds. After an aerosol exposure to a yellow rain–like attack, mycotoxins will be trapped in the nose, throat, and upper respiratory tract. If the toxin has been swallowed or inhaled, take oral superactivated charcoal. Irrigate your eyes with normal saline or water to remove toxin.

The only defense is to prevent exposure by wearing a protective mask and clothing (or topical skin protectant) during an attack. If you do have a mask, keep in mind that if you put it on at the first sighting of an incoming rocket or hostile aircraft, you should be able to substantially reduce your exposure. The Army recommends a lightweight face mask and also provides skin decontamination kits for its troops, including creams that, when applied, will protect against toxins, as well as materials to better remove the toxins afterward. You may purchase all these products from decontamination and counterterror companies listed at the back of this book. But it would be almost impossible for a civilian population to be this prepared as it went about its everyday tasks. Perhaps more practical for civilian populations is this piece of advice: Leave the area of the attack as soon as possible to limit your exposure.

If you suffer residual soreness or redness of the skin after decontamination, calamine or other lotions or creams, such as 0.25% camphor and methanol, may help. You may also suffer continued upper respiratory irritation (sore throat, hoarseness, nonproductive cough), and these may be relieved by steam inhalation, codeine or another substance to suppress the cough, and other simple measures. If respiratory symptoms are severe, however, you must do all you can to get to the hospital or seek out the treatment of a doctor skilled in respiratory care.

Please note that T-2 poisoning progresses from contact symptoms to systemic symptoms, including weakness and lack of coordination, rapidly. Clearly the latter is the more advanced and lethal disease. The Army also reports on the following preliminary research findings, which may be of use in the event of a yellow rain attack:

- High doses of systemic glucocorticosteroids, a hormone-based therapy used for asthma, seems to increase survival time "by decreasing the primary injury and the shocklike state that follows exposure to trichothecene mycotoxins."
- Platelet-activating factor can prolong the survival of rats exposed to a lethal dose of T-2 toxin.
- Dosing before and after the exposure with diphenhydramine (an antihistame) or naloxone (used for emergency resuscitation after heroin overdose) prolonged the survival times of mice exposed subcutaneously or topically with lethal doses of T-2 toxin.
- Therapy to promote detoxification and excretion of T-2, tested in

swine, combined metoclopramide, activated charcoal, magnesium sulfate, dexamethasone, sodium bicarbonate, and normal saline. All treatment groups showed improved survival times when compared with the nontreated T-2 controls.

Civilians may be especially interested in the following research finding: ascorbic acid, in other words, simple vitamin C, has been associated with enhanced chance of survival.

What You Need to Know to Survive an Attack of Yellow Rain

- Leave the area of the attack as soon as possible to limit your exposure.
- As you are leaving, cover eyes, nose, and mouth to minimize irritation.
- Do not touch anyone who has or has not been contaminated.
- Do not touch your face, since this can spread contamination to mucous membranes and worsen the course of disease.
- Outer clothing should be removed and exposed skin decontaminated with soap and water.
- Eye exposure should be treated with copious saline irrigation.
- Contact with contaminated skin and clothing can produce secondary dermal exposures. Therefore, wear gloves, mask, and gown with anyone who has been exposed until decontamination is accomplished.
- T-2 can be absorbed through intact skin. So it's critical to decontaminate as soon as possible. However, before you wash off, blot off excess material. In that way you won't spread it onto uninvolved skin.
- Decontaminate any surface that has been exposed. Environmental decontamination requires that a mixture of bleach and sodium hydrochloride remain on a surface for one hour.
- No matter what the route of delivery, T-2 has both contact effects and systemic effects. The contact effects include irritation to mucous membranes such as eyes, nose, skin, airway, and gastroin-

testinal tract. The systemic effects include weakness, bone marrow suppression, and loss of coordination. Systemic symptoms indicate full-fledged T-2 disease, and can occur rapidly after exposure.

- If you have symptoms, enter the public health pipeline as soon as possible.
- Consider purchasing a military-quality decontamination kit from a reputable counterterrorist supply company.
- Some research indicates that vitamin C can enhance your choice of survival.
- Report suspected cases of T-2 mycotoxin or suspected intentional release of yellow rain to your local health department. The local health department is responsible for notifying the state health department, the FBI, and local law enforcement. The state health department will notify the CDC.

Staphylococcal Enterotoxin B

Delivery: Aerosol or sabotage of food or water supply.

Symptoms: Headache, cough, shortness of breath, chest pain, nausea, vomiting, diarrhea, and muscle pain. Can lead to pulmonary edema, respiratory failure, and death in a small percentage of cases.

Timeline: Symptoms start 3–12 hours after inhalation or 4–10 hours after ingestion. Illness may last from hours up to 2 weeks.

Can be mistaken for: Any respiratory disease, such as influenza, mycoplasmosis, or adenovirus. Can also be mistaken for diseases with severe gastrointestinal symptoms, like cholera.

Treatment: Supportive therapy, including artificial ventilation and fluid management, and antitoxin.

SEB in Nature

Staphylococcal enterotoxin B (SEB) is excreted by the bacterium *Staphylococcus aureus,* a species known for living and reproducing in unrefrigerated meats, dairy, and bakery products. SEB causes inflammation and acts especially in the intestines, making it an enterotoxin. SEB itself is the most common cause of classic food poisoning; another toxin, also produced by the *Staphylococcus aureus* bacterium, is responsible for toxic shock syndrome.

SEB as an Agent of Biological War

SEB has been studied as a weapon of war because it can be easily aerosolized, is very stable, and can cause widespread systemic damage, multiorgan system failure, and even shock and death when inhaled at very high dosages. Classified as an incapacitating agent, SEB rarely kills. Instead it causes temporary but profound illness that incapacitates about 80% of those exposed for a week or two, potentially overwhelming the health care pipeline.

These characteristics thrust SEB onto the list of seven biological agents stockpiled by the United States during its old bioweapons program, which was terminated in 1969.

Signs and Symptoms

Symptoms of SEB intoxication begin 3–12 hours after inhalation, or 4–10 hours after ingestion. Symptoms include nonspecific flulike symptoms (fever, chills, headache, and muscle pain) and specific features dependent on the route of exposure. Oral exposure results in predominantly gastrointestinal symptoms: nausea, vomiting, and diarrhea. Inhalation exposures produce predominantly respiratory symptoms: nonproductive cough, chest pain, and shortness of breath. GI symptoms may accompany respiratory exposure due to inadvertent swallowing of the toxin.

The fever may last up to 5 days and range from 103° to 106°F, with variable degrees of chills and prostration, and cough may last for up to 4 weeks.

How Medical Professionals Diagnose SEB

Diagnosis of SEB intoxication is clinical, although it is easy to confuse with flu or many other bacterial and viral ills. Physicians will suspect SEB attack when patients present in large numbers within about 24 hours, in contrast to naturally occurring pneumonia or influenza, where patients would present over a more prolonged interval of time. Naturally occurring staphylococcal food poisoning cases would not present with pulmonary symptoms. SEB intoxication can be differentiated from more lethal infections, like anthrax or tularemia, because it generally plateaus, whereas these other infections, if untreated, tend to progress to death.

Laboratory confirmation of SEB intoxication includes blood samples for detection of antigens or environmental samples, used to analyze DNA. SEB may not be detectable in the serum by the time symptoms occur; regardless, a serum specimen should be drawn as early as possible after exposure. Data from rabbit studies clearly show that the presence of SEB in the serum is transient; however, it accumulates in the urine and can be detected for several hours postexposure. Therefore, urine samples should also be obtained and tested for SEB. Respiratory secretions and nasal swabs may demonstrate the toxin early (within 24 hours of exposure). Because most patients will develop a significant antibody response to the toxin, acute and convalescent sera should be drawn for retrospective diagnosis.

Care and Treatment

Currently, therapy is limited to supportive care. In light of this, the good news for caretakers is that SEB poisoning is not contagious. Once the victim has been decontaminated, he or she can be cared for without any worry that the illness will make others sick.

Caretakers must make sure that patients have sufficient oxygen, and that they do not become dehydrated or, on the other hand, that they do not retain excess water. Depending upon the situation, the victim may require intravenous hydration or a diuretic. Although less than 1% of victims succumb to this toxin, death, when it occurs, is due to edema (water on the lungs) or respiratory failure, so these symptoms must be addressed.

If you have oxygen in the house for a patient with a chronic condition, and if there is an extra supply, you may want to share some with the SEB patient who has trouble breathing.

It may be difficult for someone without medical training to tell the difference between the two "opposite" conditions of dehydration and water retention. Here are some tips: You may suspect dehydration if fingers turn pale and if urine is dark yellow or orangish instead of the lighter color of straw. For infants, make sure they wet diapers at the same rate, and in the same volume, as before. Dehydrated individuals have trouble producing an abundance of tears. If, by looking at these clues, you determine that an SEB-exposed patient is dehydrated, your best bet is to get the patient to the hospital for intravenous hydration—attempting this at home can place the patient at risk.

Victims should receive acetaminophen for fever, and cough suppressants for cough. Some clinicians have suggested use of steroids, but their value is unknown and thus, these are not advised. Instead, say those who have dealt with this toxin, most patients are expected to do well after the initial, acute phase of the illness, although they will need to rest for a couple of weeks.

Although there is currently no human vaccine for immunization against SEB intoxication, several candidates are in the works, and animal studies for these are promising.

What You Need to Know to Survive an Attack of SEB

- Those who die of SEB succumb to respiratory failure or edema, so fluid balance and ventilation are of the utmost importance.
- Decontamination of most surfaces may be accomplished with soap and water or with exposure to household bleach.
- Foods that may have been contaminated should be destroyed.
- Protective masks such as those employed by military units offer excellent protection for those individuals alert to the possibility of attack.
- Antibiotics are of no benefit, and no antitoxin has been developed.
- SEB is inactivated after a few minutes at 100°F.

14

Ricin

Ricin in Nature

Ricin is a toxic protein derived from the beans of the castor plant (*Ricinus communis*), which is ubiquitous worldwide. Because the toxin is easy to extract and prepare, ricin can be spread with virtually no special equipment and little technical knowledge or skill. What it lacks in complexity, moreover, it makes up for with venom: this poison is particularly cruel, inhibiting DNA reproduction and protein synthesis, the drivers of life, so that victims will die some 36 hours after symptoms begin.

Though castor beans have long been valued for their therapeutic power, people have understood their dark side since ancient times. The beans were cultivated in Egypt for the lubricating and laxative effects of their oil. That oil was also used to lubricate aircraft in both World War I and World War II.

But when producers extracted the good from castor beans, they left the poison behind. The toxin, which remains in the castor meal after the oil has been removed, is itself extracted through a simple "salting-out" procedure. In 1888, a German researcher identified the toxin as a protein he named ricin.

Less than a decade later, the founder of immunology, Paul Ehrlich, used his study of ricin to demonstrate the immune response. Feeding mice and rabbits with small amounts of the castor seeds, Ehrlich was able to induce immunity to ricin, proving that when appropriately stimulated the blood could generate "antibodies"—proteins able to neutralize invading germs.

While researchers still have not successfully developed a ricin vaccine based on these findings, they have used the toxin's destructive power to positive end. In the 1950s, other scientists showed the toxic protein could inhibit tumor growth. Today, as an extension of that work, ricin is part of the arsenal of anticancer drugs with the potential to heal.

Ricin as a Weapon of Biological Terror

It only makes sense that when the United States started stocking its armory of biological weapons, ricin—so toxic and yet so simple to produce—would be a choice. Code-named Compound W, ricin was studied by the U.S. Chemical Warfare Service in collaboration with the British at the end of World War I. That joint effort resulted in development of the "W Bomb," a weapon that experts say was tested but never used.

Ricin *was* used, however, in the infamous Cold War assassination of Bulgarian dissident and defector Georgi Markov, who worked as an announcer for Radio Free Europe in London before his murder in 1978. Markov's murder was so bizarrely futuristic, it could have been part of a plot in a James Bond flick.

In fact, it was. In the 1981 film *For Your Eyes Only* James Bond's quartermaster, Major Boothroyd (a.k.a. Q) sported a lethal umbrella with hidden metal hooks that sprang into action and closed on a victim's neck when triggered. The filmmakers may have taken their cue from the Bulgarian Secret Service and the KGB: Markov's assassins, too, used a weapon disguised as an umbrella—a gun rigged to deliver a pellet containing a few hundred millionths of a gram of ricin, supplied by the KGB. Sneaking up on Markov, agents were able to use their umbrella gun to inject the toxin into Markov's thigh.

Speaking at the inquest after the murder, Markov's wife described the scene: "He told me that while waiting for a bus on the south side of Waterloo Bridge he had felt a jab in the back of his right thigh and, looking around, saw a man drop an umbrella. The man said he was sorry and Georgi said that he got the impression that he was trying to cover his face as he rushed off and hailed a taxi.

"Georgi told me he thought the man must have been a foreigner because the taxi driver seemed to have some difficulty in understanding him. He showed me some blood on his jeans and a mark like a puncture, about the size of the tip of a ballpoint pen on the back of his right thigh."

The next day, she took him to the hospital, where he experienced a gruesome descent through illness to death. Thirty-six hours after the incident, Markov had fever, rapid heartbeat, and swollen lymph nodes in the groin. At 48 hours his blood pressure plummeted, his pulse soared, his cardiovascular system collapsed, and he went into shock. By day three he had stopped urinating and started vomiting blood. An electrocardiogram demonstrated complete blockage of his blood vessels, and shortly thereafter he died.

According to U.S. intelligence, this was just the first of seven similar attacks, many of them successful, using ricin injected by pellet gun. But while ricin was a favorite tool of the "I Spy" set, it was also gaining popularity among a more local crowd.

If there is a single bioweapon that might qualify as the "poor man's poison," ricin is it. While other agents require scientific sophistication and, often, industrial-quality production lines, ricin is so simple to prepare it is even covered in "how-to" murder manuals like *The Poisoner's Handbook, Silent Death,* and the cult favorite, *Catalogue of Silent Tools of Justice*, currently out of print. Before PCs were common, and long before instructions for making nuclear bombs were posted through the Internet, ricin recipes were easy to find.

Ease of use has thrust ricin to the top of the weapons list for individuals involved in extremist movements, as well as those who, for whatever reason, seek to cause another harm. Those involved in recent ricin incidents include:

- Two tax protesters from a group called the Minnesota Patriot's Council, convicted of possessing ricin as a biological weapon in February 1995, constituting the first case of prosecution under the 1989 Biological Weapons Anti-Terrorism Act.
- A retired electrician who had worked the trans-Alaska pipeline and was arrested in 1993 after Canadian customs officials found his car loaded with guns, 20,000 rounds of ammunition, neo-Nazi literature, instruction manuals for chemical and biological weapons— oh, and a bag full of ricin. He told authorities he was preparing to control the coyote problem on his farm.
- A Kansas City oncologist who, in 1996, pleaded guilty to poisoning her cardiologist husband with ricin toxin—three times! Though he became severely ill, he recovered after each attack because despite her best efforts, she failed to deliver a sufficient dose.

The destructive power of ricin has apparently impressed al Qaeda terrorists in Afghanistan. In a front-page report in the *Times* of London, the paper's correspondent in Kabul, Anthony Lloyd, said he found instructions on how to manufacture the lethal toxin in the cellar of an abandoned house used by al Qaeda members. "A strong dose will be able to kill an adult and a dose equal to seven seeds will kill a child," one page of instructions read. Another page read: "Gloves and face mask are essential for the preparation of ricin. Period of death varies from 3–5 days minimum, 4–14 days maximum."

Lloyd reported it was unclear whether al Qaeda members had ever actually produced ricin toxin, like the Bulgarian secret police before. It may be difficult to learn the truth: The two Arab doctors who worked in the facility where the ricin was discovered were beaten to death as they tried to escape. No ricin-injecting umbrellas were found.

Signs and Symptoms

Specific symptoms as well as the outcome depend upon the route of exposure and the intensity of the dose. In the 1940s, when a group of individuals were accidentally exposed to a sublethal dose of aerosolized toxin, they developed fever, chest tightness, cough, shortness of breath, nausea, and joint pain 4–8 hours after the accident occurred. Profuse sweating hours later signaled that the attack was over. The symptoms subsided, and those exposed got well.

Lethal exposure to aerosolized ricin leads to severe respiratory symptoms and a painful, rapid death. Patients would progress from respiratory distress to respiratory failure and finally, multiorgan failure. The toxin would cause these patients to bleed to death as diffuse hemorraging increased and blood flowed from the body's pores.

If ingested, ricin causes severe gastrointestinal symptoms, ranging from nausea and abdominal pain to internal bleeding and death.

If injected, ricin toxin affects muscles first, but multiorgan failure is the endpoint here, as well.

How Medical Professionals Diagnose Ricin

If large numbers of patients from a single geographic area report to the emergency department with severe damage to the lungs, ricin could be the cause. The medical suspicion would intensify if antibiotics failed to ease the symptoms, and if the patients progressed to shock, organ failure, and death within 36 hours of the time they took ill. This extremely rapid decline would be unusual, indeed, with exposure to bacterial or viral disease. While any differential diagnosis would need to include SEB, Q fever, tularemia, and plague, only ricin would tend to cause so much death so fast.

Laboratory diagnosis would not help in the event of acute symptoms from ricin, since the illness would progress faster than tests could be performed. Nonetheless, physicians hoping to confirm the diagnosis after the fact would send serum or respiratory secretions to a lab for analysis. If ricin is the cause, antigens in the blood should be found. A polymerase chain reaction test would detect castor bean DNA in samples from the environment.

Care and Treatment

There is no medication, antitoxin, or vaccine available for ricin poisoning today. The best protection against this deadly toxin is use of a protective mask, but unfortunately, one would have to have advance warning of attack for the mask to work. If ricin or other toxins and chemicals are of concern to you, you might carry a simple, paper surgical mask in your pocket or briefcase. Of course, it won't do you much good unless you have been able to predict the attack in advance, unlikely with a weapon whose strength is covert action.

If you have been exposed to the toxin, remove your outer clothing on the spot and vacate the area. Then shower with soap and shampoo as rapidly as possibly to mitigate the severity of your symptoms. Hypochlorite solutions (0.1% sodium hypochlorite) can inactivate ricin. The victim should drink plenty of fluids to deal with fluid loss, but if he or she is clinically dehydrated, you will need the aid of a hospital or clinic established to deal with this issue intravenously. Rehydrating a ricin patient without emergency medical backup can be risky.

The mainstay of care for the ricin victim is support, almost always at a hospital. If the toxin has been inhaled, pulmonary symptoms can be treated with oxygen, intubation, or artificial ventilation. If the poison has been ingested, the stomach may need to be pumped and then vomiting induced. At the emergency department, physicians might use superactivated charcoal to absorb the toxin, followed by use of cathartics such as magnesium citrate. They would also replace fluids through intravenous hydration. This is beyond what the individual can do at home—call your local poison control center and request that help be sent.

What You Need to Know to Survive an Attack of Ricin

- The best defense against aerosolized ricin toxin is a face mask—but only if you are aware of the attack as it is ongoing. If the attack is covert, a face mask won't be much help.
- If you have been caught up in an attack, remove your outer clothes and vacate the area. Then shower with soap, shampoo, and water as soon as possible.

- Use hypochlorite solutions (0.1% sodium hypochlorite) to inactivate ricin.
- Get to a hospital, especially if you think you may be dehydrated. Because of the complexity of the response, rehydrating a dehydrated victim can be dangerous outside a hospital or other facility equipped for emergency medical response.
- Get to a hospital so pulmonary complications can be treated with ventilation.
- If you believe a ricin attack may be or has been attempted, alert local law enforcement at once.

CONCLUSION
Family Preparedness

Can we ever really prepare for a catastrophic outbreak of bioterrorism? If terrorists succeed in causing widespread infection with smallpox, Ebola, or the plague, what can we do to improve our chance of making it through?

The very effort might feel futile. By its very nature, after all, a biological attack is covert. It will be almost impossible to recognize the attack until hours, days, or weeks after it has occurred.

If you happen to be at ground zero (the location where the weapon is released) or if you are patient zero (first to come down with the disease) then your chance of survival may, in fact, be slim. But in the event of catastrophic infection, chances are overwhelmingly high that you will not be part of these unfortunate groups. In fact, in any wide-scale assault, most of those who succumb will be in the second wave of victims or beyond. In this instance, even given the collapse of the social structure, there is plenty you can to do improve your chance of survival.

If there is one piece of advice for anyone caught up in a bioterrorist assault, it is this: If the government comes through with the resources of the health care pipeline, if you have access to hospitals, clinics, doctors, and experts, go with the flow. Let government-provided physicians treat you with government-stockpiled medication in official facilities. Do not, under any circumstance, attempt to take care of yourself or direct your own treatment when you have access to the staff, the medical protocols, and the resources of official help. If official help is available to you, you are fortunate, indeed.

The fear of many, of course, is that catastrophic assault will cause the health care pipeline to shut down. Should an attack victimize tens of thousands, possibly millions, of Americans, the thinking goes, hospitals will be overwhelmed and understaffed, or perhaps unavailable at all. Should you want to go elsewhere for help, moreover, highways could be clogged with traffic, or possibly blocked by military units in hazmat suits charged with quarantining the infected and exposed, thus containing the disease. Stockpiles of needed medications could be depleted within days, depending upon the specific drug needed, or perhaps just unavailable. If the corner pharmacist has locked up shop and fled the scene of infection, you may be unable to obtain medication for your sick child. Supermarkets and hardware stores may be closed, and public services across a range of areas, from transportation to energy to telephone, may function sporadically or not at all. Police and fire services may be severely compromised, and the continuity of government itself over wide geographic regions may be temporarily broken.

Under such circumstances, each family will be on its own, with the ability to survive the outbreak dependent upon the thoroughness of preparation—including level of knowledge about the biological agent itself—before the attack occurred. In such an instance, the level of preparedness you establish now could indeed determine whether or not you make it through.

General Disaster Management: A Red Cross Primer for Families

Many of the things you must do to prepare are not specific to a bioterrorism disaster, but might equally apply to catastrophic earthquakes, hurricanes, or floods. Experts often suggest that you have supplies on hand to sustain yourself for a few days to a week. While quarantines can last up to 3 weeks, you should reasonably expect to store a week's worth of supplies for a bioterrorist disaster as well.

What do you need? The Red Cross, the Federal Emergency

Management Agency, and many other organizations have released detailed instructions, the most relevant of them emphasized below. First, experts list the supplies and materials you need to store and gather in advance, suggesting that 6 to 12 weeks of the following be kept in reserve:

Water You must store an extra week's worth of water for each member of your family. Make sure to provide extra quantities for children and pregnant women. Each adult family member will require 2 gallons of water a day—1 gallon for drinking and food preparation, and another gallon for cleanliness, including modified showers or baths, washing dishes, and washing clothes. An average consumption of water per person, per day is 1 gallon. There are many ways to store all this water in the event of an emergency—even in a stopped-up bathtub or in 2-liter soda bottles that you have rinsed out and saved. If you buy bottled water in advance, remember that you cannot keep it indefinitely without bacteria accumulating. To prevent this, safeguard your water by adding four drops of scent-free bleach to each 2-liter bottle of water. Make certain that you use regular household bleach, and stay away from formulations of the high-chlorine variety. If you use water from a bathtub, be sure to boil it before consumption. If you plan to use commercially prepared "spring" or "drinking" water, keep the water in its original sealed container. Change and replace the water at least once a year. Once opened, use it and do not store it further. For the cost of about $200 or $300, you may even consider purchasing a water purifier.

Food As with water, you will need at least a 1-week supply to prepare adequately. You must attend to this now, not after the attack has occurred—after all, supermarkets tend to stock only a few days of goods, and everyone will have the same idea as you in the event of a catastrophe. Find a cool, dark place for this extra food, which should be selected for durability and shelf life. Keep in mind that you can keep canned food for about two years. Also worth considering are dehydrated, freeze-dried foods, which are available from camping stores or catalogs. While costly, these items have a shelf life of 10–15 years. Continue to use food from the stockpile and replace it with new food so that, in essence, you are renewing stored food every 6 months.

Communication   Make sure you have a couple of transistor radios with a plentiful supply of batteries. A laptop computer with wireless Internet and a cell phone are also advisable, although it is anyone's guess as to whether or not these utilities will work.

Transportation   Try to see to it that your family vehicles are filled with gasoline on a regular basis.

Medication   Make sure you are stocked up on nonprescription medications, including aspirin or nonaspirin pain reliever and anti-inflammatory drug, antidiarrhea treatments, laxative, antacid (for stomach upset), and syrup of ipecac and activated charcoal, both for use only by instruction of the Poison Control Center. Also, make sure you have an extra month's supply of any medication you take for chronic conditions, from heart disease to depression. In any disaster, especially involving biological agents, your local drugstore and the health delivery system in general could be severely compromised and dysfunctional, or even nonfunctional, for a period of time.

First Aid   Spend some time now in purchasing or putting together a comprehensive first aid kit along with an instruction book to administer first aid in an emergency. Assemble a first aid kit for your home and one for each car. Among the supplies you should have: sterile adhesive bandages in assorted sizes; assorted sizes of safety pins; cleansing agent/soap; latex gloves (2 pairs); sunscreen; 2-inch sterile gauze pads (4–6 per kit); 4-inch sterile gauze pads (4–6 per kit); triangular bandages (3 per kit); 2-inch sterile roller bandages (3 rolls per kit); 3-inch sterile roller bandages (3 rolls per kit); scissors, tweezers, and needle; moistened towelettes; antiseptic; thermometer; tongue blades (2 per kit); and a tube of petroleum jelly or other lubricant.

Cash   After a disaster, you may need cash for the first few days, or even several weeks. Income may stop if you can't work. To help stay solvent, keep a small amount of cash or traveler's checks at home in a place where you can get at it quickly in case of a sudden evacuation. A disaster can shut down local ATMs and banks. The money should be in small denominations for easier use. Consider also opening a small, fluid bank account outside your local area, since a disaster that affects you could also affect your local financial institutions.

Preparing a Disaster Kit

You must prepare an emergency disaster kit that you may use at home or take with you should you need to evacuate. All items in the kit should be placed in a sturdy suitcase with wheels, a duffel bag, or a large, covered plastic garbage pail (also with rollers). The kit should include:

Tools and Supplies   Mess kits or paper cups, plates, and plastic utensils; a battery-operated radio and a few flashlights with plenty of extra batteries; cash or traveler's checks, as well as change, preferably quarters; a nonelectric can opener and utility knife; fire extinguisher; tube tent; pliers; tape; compass; matches in a waterproof container; aluminum foil; plastic storage containers; signal flare; paper and writing utensils; needles and thread; medicine dropper; shutoff wrench, to turn off household gas and water; whistle; plastic sheeting; map of the area (for locating shelters); plastic garbage bags; and duct tape.

Sanitation Materials   Toilet paper, moist towelettes; soap; liquid detergent; a plastic bucket with a tight lid; disinfectant; and household chlorine bleach.

Clothing and Bedding   At least one complete change of clothing and footwear per person. Sturdy shoes or work boots, rain gear, blankets or sleeping bags, and outerwear for cold weather, including thermal underwear, hat, and gloves.

Important Family Documents   Make copies of all essential documents and store them elsewhere, in a location outside your home and, ideally, outside of your specific city or region. In addition, store another set of documents in a waterproof container or protective plastic bag in your home. You should include insurance policies, contracts, proof of residence including deeds, recent tax returns, wills, power of attorney, stocks and bonds or records of them, passports, Social Security cards, bank account numbers, credit card account numbers and companies. Also: inventory of valuable household goods, important telephone numbers, and birth, marriage, and death certificates. Make sure that you do not evacuate without your driver's license or personal identification.

Medical Records Immunizations, x-rays, charts. Anything you have to document your health status.

Keep a smaller version of the supplies from the disaster kit in the trunk of each car that you own. Among the items to include: battery-operated radio, a couple of flashlights with spare bulbs and batteries, several six-packs of bottled water, a few compressed food bars or candy bars, and a first aid kit. That should be enough to keep a family of four going for up to a day—no need to prepare the car for weeks on the run.

Disaster Action Plan

In addition to things you must have, the Red Cross says, there are things you must do:

A Safe Room Pick an upstairs room, because nerve gas and other toxic gases and mists are often heavier than air, settling at ground level. (*Note:* For other disasters, including hurricane or tornado, the safe room might be appropriately prepared on a lower level, or even in a basement.) Stash a couple of rolls of duct tape and plastic sheeting or trash bags in the room to seal around doors and windows and to close off heating and air conditioning ducts. This is a good place to store your family disaster kit, since it is the place where you will use it if you are asked to "shelter in place." Make sure that you have, stored in this safe room, a transistor radio with plenty of batteries, as well as food and water. Do not come out of the safe room until the radio instructs you that it is safe to do so.

An Emergency Communications Plan Choose an out-of-town contact your family or household will call or e-mail to check on each other should a disaster occur. Your selected contact should live far enough away that they would be unlikely to be directly affected by the same event, and they should know they are the chosen contact. Make sure every household member has that contact's, and each other's, e-mail addresses and telephone numbers (home, work, pager, and cell). Leave these contact numbers at your children's schools, if you have children, and at your workplace. Your family should know that if telephones are not working, they need to be patient and try again later or try e-mail. Many people flood the telephone lines when emergencies happen, but e-mail can sometimes get through when calls don't. Make sure that every individual in your family, especially the children, always have enough change to make a phone call. Make sure you teach your children how to reverse the charges.

Your Children's Schools   If you have children, check with their schools to make sure you are thoroughly aware of emergency plans. Ask in advance what you will need to do to authorize the pickup of your child by someone other than yourself; the school may be unreachable by phone during the emergency itself. Have your own plan as to how all your children will get home as rapidly as possible.

Your Community   Stay in touch with your community. Learn about your community's warning signals—what they sound like and what you should do.

Evacuation   Listen to your radio or television and follow the instructions of local emergency officials. If you are asked to evacuate, do so immediately—there is probably good reason for the request. Even if it is summer, wear clothing that is protective, including long-sleeved shirts, long pants, and sturdy shoes. Take your disaster supplies kit. Take your pets with you; do not leave them behind, or you may find you will not be allowed back to care for them. (See page 177 for specific advice on pet care.) Be sure to use travel routes specified by local authorities—don't use shortcuts, because certain areas may be impassable or dangerous. Remember, if local authorities ask you to leave your home, they have a good reason, and you should heed the advice immediately. If you have time, call your family contact to tell them where you will be going.

Special note: The Red Cross says that if you are advised by local officials to "shelter in place," what they mean is for you to remain inside your home or office and protect yourself there. Close and lock all windows and exterior doors. Turn off all fans and heating and air conditioning systems. Close the fireplace damper. Get your disaster supplies kit, and make sure the radio is working. Go to an interior room without windows that's above ground level (your safe room). In the case of a chemical threat, an above-ground location is preferable because some chemicals are heavier than air, and may seep into basements even if the windows are closed. Keep listening to your radio or television until you are told all is safe or you are told to evacuate. Have maps in the car so that you do not get lost.

Food and Water on the Fly

It's not a pleasant thought, but what if, in the face of sudden attack, you have not yet gathered your supplies or made your preparations? What if all you have to help you "shelter in place" is this book? In that case, take note that you can access water from the environment, or even the pipes in your home.

For water, the Red Cross suggests you look to rain, streams, rivers, and other moving bodies, including natural springs. Avoid water with floating material, an odor, or a dark color. That said, if a pond or lake is clear, you may tap that source as well. No matter where you get the water, make sure that you treat it as instructed on the following pages before drinking.

You can also find hidden supplies of usable water in your office building or home, in such niches as your hot-water tank and pipes, and even the ice cubes in your freezer. As a last resort, you can use water in the reservoir tank of your toilet (not the bowl).

To use the water in your pipes, let air into the plumbing by turning on the faucet in your house at the highest level. A small amount of water will trickle out. Then obtain water from the lowest faucet in the house. To use the water in your hot-water tank, be sure the electricity or gas is off, and open the drain at the bottom of the tank. Start the water flowing by turning off the water intake valve and turning on a hot-water faucet. Do not turn on the gas or electricity when the tank is empty.

The Red Cross also advises that you treat water with any potential for contamination for any reason. This is most urgent in the wake of terrorist attacks, since contamination of the water supply may be part of the perpetrators' strategic plan. Contaminated water can carry cholera, dysentery, typhoid, hepatitis, and any number of other debilitating or lethal germs, as covered in the chapters of this book. Contaminated water will sometimes have a bad odor or taste; other times it will seem to be healthy and clean.

Treat all water of uncertain purity with at least one of the following methods, and preferably, a combination of at least two:

Boiling Bring water to a rolling boil for 3–5 minutes, keeping in mind that some water will evaporate. Let the water cool before drinking. Boiled water will taste better if you put oxygen back into it by pouring the water back and forth between two clean containers. This will also improve the taste of stored water.

Disinfection Use household liquid bleach to kill microorganisms. Use only regular household liquid bleach that contains 5.25% sodium hypochlorite; avoid products with higher concentrations. Do not use scented bleaches, colorsafe bleaches, or bleaches with added cleaners. Add 4 drops of bleach to each 2-liter bottle of water (as many as 16 drops of bleach per gallon of water is fine). Stir and let the water stand for half an hour. If the water does not have a slight bleach odor, repeat the dosage and let stand another 15 minutes.

Distillation Boiling and disinfection will remove germs but these methods are unable to treat heavy metals, salts, and most chemicals. To deal with these issues, water must be distilled. This is more complex but will provide you greater protection against contamination. Distillation involves boiling water and then collecting the vapor that condenses back to water. The condensed vapor will not include salt and other impurities. A procedure outlined by the Red Cross can work well in the home: Make sure you have a sizable pot with a secure lid. Fill the pot halfway with water. Tie a cup to the handle on the pot's lid so that the cup will hang right side up when the lid is upside down (make sure the cup is not dangling into the water) and boil the water for 20 minutes. The water that drips from the lid into the cup is distilled. This is time consuming, but if your family drinks only distilled water, you will be far less likely to get sick from anything terrorists might do to the water supply. If you treat distilled water with bleach, you should be extremely well protected.

Straining You will have even greater protection if you strain water through layers of paper towels or clean cloths before treating, as a means of removing contaminants involving larger particles.

Finally, if your water supply is limited, stay away from salty foods, as well as those high in fat and protein. If the food supply itself is limited, take note that all (except for growing children and pregnant women) can get by on half the normal amount of calories by reducing their activity.

Basic Disaster Supplies Kit Checklist

The Red Cross suggests that you use the following checklist to make sure you have all supplies needed for your disaster kit. Keep in mind that in the event of a catastrophic biological attack, you may need to purchase provisions below for a time period ranging from 6 to 12 weeks.

Essentials
____Battery-operated radio and extra batteries
____Flashlight and extra batteries
Do not include candles. Candles cause more fires after a disaster than anything else.

Water
Store water in plastic containers, such as large soft drink bottles. Avoid using containers that will decompose or break, such as milk cartons or glass bottles. A person who is generally active needs to drink at least 2 quarts of water each day. Hot environments and intense physical activity can double that amount. Children, nursing mothers, and ill people will need to drink even more. Store three gallons of water per person (1 gallon for each day and for each person). Keep at least a 3-day supply of water (2 quarts for drinking, 2 quarts for food preparation and sanitation) for each person in the household.

Food
Store at least a 3-day supply of nonperishable food. Select foods that require no refrigeration, preparation, or cooking and little or no

(continued)

water. If you must heat food, pack a can of Sterno and water-proof matches. Select food items that are compact and lightweight. Include a selection of the following foods in your disaster supplies kit:

____Ready-to-eat canned fish, such as tuna.
____Canned fruits, dried fruits, and nuts
____Canned vegetables

First Aid Kit

Assemble a first aid kit for your home and one for each car. A first aid kit should include the following:

____Sterile, adhesive bandages in assorted sizes
____Assorted sizes of safety pins
____Cleansing agent/soap
____Latex gloves (2 pairs)
____Sunscreen
____2-inch sterile gauze pads (4–6)
____4-inch sterile gauze pads (4–6)
____Triangular bandages (3)
____2-inch sterile roller bandages (3 rolls)
____3-inch sterile roller bandages (3 rolls)
____Scissors
____Adhesive tape
____Tweezers
____Needle
____Moistened towelettes
____Antiseptic
____Rubbing alcohol
____Thermometer
____Tongue blades (2)
____Tube of petroleum jelly or other lubricant
____Extra eyeglasses

Nonprescription Drugs

____Aspirin or nonaspirin pain reliever
____Antidiarrheal medication
____Antacid (for stomach upset)
____Syrup of ipecac (use to induce vomiting if advised by the Poison Control Center)

____Laxative

____Activated charcoal (use if advised by the Poison Control Center)

Sanitation

____Toilet paper, towelettes

____Soap, liquid detergent

____Feminine hygiene supplies

____Personal hygiene items

____Plastic garbage bags, ties (for personal sanitation uses)

____Plastic bucket with tight lid

____Disinfectant

____Household chlorine bleach (use only regular household liquid bleach that contains 5.25% sodium hypochlorite)

____Facial tissues

____Condoms

Clothing and Bedding

____One complete change of clothing and footwear per person

____Sturdy shoes or work boots

____Rain gear

____Blankets or sleeping bags

____Hat and gloves

____Thermal underwear

____Sunglasses

Tools and Supplies

____Mess kits or paper cups; plates and plastic utensils

____Cash or traveler's checks, coins

____Nonelectric can opener, utility knife

____Pliers, screwdriver, hammer, crowbar, assorted nails, wood screws

____Shutoff wrench, to turn off household gas and water

____Tape, such as duct tape

____Compass

____Matches in a waterproof container

____Aluminum foil

____Plastic storage containers

(continued)

_____Signal flare
_____Paper, pencil
_____Needles, thread
_____Medicine dropper
_____Adhesive labels
_____Safety goggles
_____Heavy work gloves
_____Whistle
_____Heavy cotton or hemp rope
_____Patch kit and can of seal-in-air
_____Videocassettes
_____Disposable dust masks
_____Plastic sheeting
_____Map of the area (for locating shelters)

For Baby
_____Formula
_____Diapers/wipes
_____Bottles
_____Powdered formula, milk, or baby food
_____Medications

Important Family Documents
Keep these records in a waterproof, portable container:

_____Copy of will, insurance policies, contracts, deeds, stocks and bonds
_____Copy of passports, Social Security cards, immunization records
_____Record of credit card accounts
_____Record of bank account numbers, names, and phone numbers
_____Inventory of valuable household goods, important telephone numbers
_____Family records (birth, marriage, death certificates)
_____Copy of Supplemental Security Income award letter

Medical Needs
_____Heart and high blood pressure medication
_____Insulin

_____Prescription drugs
_____Denture supplies
_____Contact lenses and supplies

Items for Service Animals/Pets
(Remember, if you wind up in a Red Cross shelter, your pets will not be allowed, so do make alternate provisions for them ahead of time.)

_____Food
_____Additional water
_____Collar
_____Leash/harness
_____Identification tags
_____Medications, vaccinations and medical records
_____Litter/pan

Entertainment
_____Games, books, and child's favorite toy.

Other Disaster Supplies
Assemble the supplies below in addition to your basic disaster supplies kit. Combine these with your disaster supplies kit as you need them, and store them in a convenient location.

Disability-Related Supplies and Special Equipment
Check items you use, and describe item type and location.

_____Glasses:
_____Eating utensils:
_____Grooming utensils:
_____Dressing devices:
_____Writing devices:
_____Hearing device:
_____Oxygen:

Flow rate:
_____Suction equipment:
_____Dialysis equipment:
_____Sanitary supplies:
_____Urinary supplies:
_____Ostomy supplies:
_____Wheelchair:

(continued)

Wheelchair repair kit:

Motorized:

Manual:
____Walker:
____Crutches:
____Cane(s):
____Dentures:
____Monitors:
____Other:

Portable Disaster Supplies Kit
____Emergency information list/other lists
____Small flashlight
____Whistle/other noisemaker
____Water
____Extra medication
____Copies of prescriptions
____Extra pair of eyeglasses
____Hearing aid
____Sanitary supplies
____Pad and pencil or other writing device

Car Supplies
____Several blankets
____Extra set of mittens or gloves, wool socks, and a wool cap
____Jumper cables and instructions
____Small sack of sand or kitty litter for traction
____Small shovel
____Set of tire chains or traction mats
____Red cloth to use as a flag
____CB radio or cellular telephone

For disasters of the bioterrorist kind, you can add:
____Surgical face masks (disposable HEPA masks are best, but they
       will not provide ultimate protection unless you have them fitted)
____Latex gloves
____Protective caps and gowns
____Hospital scrubs

Preparing for a Biological Attack

Preparing for a biological attack requires strategies beyond those invoked for surviving hurricanes and floods. The most important tool you have in the face of biological war may be education: a basic understanding of how to recognize and, most important, deal with a biological attack. In that sense, simply reading and familiarizing yourself with the information in this book will be a big help.

Remember, it is difficult to defend against a biological attack ahead of time because, by its very nature, it is covert. The attack will occur invisibly, under your nose—and the attackers will likely disappear into the mist long before you know that an attack has occurred. Even when people start to get sick, experts may not recognize the problem as terrorism until large numbers of patients with flulike illness progress to symptoms of Ebola, Q fever, or plague.

Dr. Paul Rega suggests that health care professionals distinguish bioterrorist activity from normal disease through the following clues:

- Severe disease in previously healthy people
- Higher than normal number of patients with fever and respiratory and/or gastrointestinal complaints
- Multiple people with similar complaints from a common location
- Endemic disease appearing at an unusual time of year
- Unusual number of rapidly fatal cases
- Greater number of ill or dead animals
- Rapidly rising and falling numbers of those swept into the epidemic
- Greater number of patients with:
  1. Severe pneumonia
  2. Sepsis (a serious infection caused by germs that overwhelm the immune system and spread throughout the body)
  3. Fever with rash
  4. Diplopia (double vision) with progressive weakness

One act of self-defense is simply to monitor your health. If you develop fever, chills, headache, and nausea stay alert, especially if the illness does not start to improve within days. If you develop symptoms you have never seen with the flu, do go to your doctor or the emergency department and check it out.

Because so many weaponized germs present, at first, as flu, more-over, getting a flu shot will not only protect you from an illness that is serious on its own, but also remove a possible source of confusion. In the event that terrorists deploy a biological weapon, reducing the likeli-hood that you will get flu makes it easier to diagnose other infections, should they occur. According to Mohammad Akhter, M.D., executive di-rector of the American Public Health Association, if you suffer flulike symptoms despite a flu shot, an educated doctor will be more likely to order blood or other tests for more exotic or unusual conditions.

Dr. Rega cautions that "it's more likely that a person with flulike symptoms who got a flu shot will have some other innocuous ailment instead of anthrax or plague." In the end, he notes, a biological attack can best be diagnosed on the community level—and the presence of many others with similar timing of unusual symptoms will be far more telling than whether or not you have gotten a shot for flu.

The Stockpiling Controversy

When it comes to bioterrorism, several issues raise the ire of experts, pitting frightened citizens against the establishment and lay people against medical professionals in what some consider matters of life and death.

Chief among the controversial issues is the question of whether indi-viduals ought to be stockpiling antibiotics like Cipro against the possi-bility that an act of bioterrorism might shut down the public health care pipeline and prevent appropriate treatments from getting through. Clearly, officials cannot sanction this kind of stockpiling, which, if done en masse, would create a medication shortage in the event of a true dis-aster. Such individual stockpiling might mean that critical medications sit in some medicine cabinets, unused, and unavailable to infected indi-viduals who may then go without treatment and die. From this perspec-tive, personal antibiotic stockpiling is seen as the ultimate selfish act.

Experts also fear that people might misuse the drugs, taking them when they have a simple cold or other illness not even responsive to an-tibiotics. Those who stockpile and then use the antibiotics when they don't need them would generate resistance to the very germs they will need to combat up the road. This would be especially dangerous in the event of a smallpox attack. Although smallpox is a virus, and thus unresponsive to antibiotics, the sick may develop debilitating secondary bacterial infections. If these individuals have been taking antibiotics all along, they may find these medications don't work against these microbes when they need them most.

What's more, a biological attack could take myriad forms, with some medications working for one agent but not another. Specific medications and combinations of medications must be prescribed and calibrated by a physician or they could either backfire or fail to help.

It bears repeating that if you have access to the public health care pipeline, you should use it. Doctors and nurses empowered by the Centers for Disease Control or your state health department will be best trained to deliver the correct medications over the correct time period at the correct dose. They will be the most valuable survival tool you have.

This said, we all must accept the possibility that health care delivery may be hampered in the hours, days, and even weeks following an attack. While you do not want to treat yourself or loved ones inappropriately, and while you do not want to hoard antibiotics, you still need to consider how you might obtain the needed medication should official emergency efforts falter or even fail.

The first thing you should do in this regard, says emergency physician Paul Rega, author of *Bio-Terry,* the stat manual for emergency rooms, is contact your personal physician for a blunt discussion about a potential action plan in the face of a catastrophic event. Should there be an attack, how can you contact your doctor to obtain medication? Will he or she be reachable by phone in the evenings? On weekends? Does your doctor have antibiotic samples or supplies at the office, or the hospital? It is important that you work out a strategy with your personal physician so that you can be taken care of if the public health care pipeline has delayed response in the aftermath of an attack.

Of course, you may be able to fill your doctor's prescription at the local pharmacy. But following a cataclysmic event, it is possible that pharmacies may be out of supplies, or unable to open at all. What if your pharmacist has fled the state, or even the country, to avoid getting ill? Keep in mind that if one pharmacy says it is out of a medication, another may be well stocked. Different chains have different arrangements with the different manufacturers, and thus have different levels of access to different drugs.

If you are unable to obtain the medication your doctor prescribes locally, you may want to try your luck by looking further afield. Can you get to a pharmacy in a different city, a different state? Can you order drugs by mail? If that fails, do you know how to purchase needed medicines from a reputable pharmacy in Mexico, in Canada, or elsewhere overseas? Clearly, in the even of a bioterrorist attack, time will be of the essence, and depending upon the weapon in question, waiting even a few days may mean the difference between life and death.

The bottom line is this: while national authorities and most health care experts object strongly to citizens' maintaining small supplies of antibiotics in the home, every individual case is different. Some individuals may be more vulnerable than others to the onslaught of infection due to personal health issues from chronic asthma to heart disease, from old age to immune dysfunction, up to and including HIV and AIDS. While public health experts advise against personal antibiotic stockpiling *in general,* they are unable to address exceptions to the rule. The truth is that your status regarding medication in the home is one you will need to determine with the help of your personal physician, the medical expert who knows you best. Your doctor will know your specific vulnerabilities and issues, and it is your doctor—not policy makers who do not know you—who is best equipped to decide whether the risk you face from possible misuse of antibiotics will be greater than the risk you could face from receiving medication only after a delay, or not obtaining it at all.

Many people, after hearing the advice of public health experts, have decided to disregard it, throwing caution to the wind and stockpiling small quantities of antibiotics in their homes; news reports note that prescriptions for Cipro in New York City are up by 600% over normal use. In most of these cases, say pharmacists, physicians have decided to write the prescriptions despite official advice. Other individuals have small quantities of antibiotics left over from previous illnesses, and have simply not bothered to throw them out. These medications sit in the medicine cabinet, and if they have not passed their expiration date, they may be tapped.

This book advises *against* stockpiling medication not specifically prescribed by a doctor treating you for the condition at hand. According to Dr. Paul Rega, the appropriate source of antibiotics following terrorist attack is the public health pipeline and the first responders who have been trained and authorized to treat the sick.

Nonetheless, if you are saving used or stockpiled antibiotics in the event that terrorists attack, you need some cautionary advice:

- Do not use any medication if it is past its expiration date, as weakened antibiotics can simply breed stronger, more resistant infections. Instead, once medications have passed the expiration date, throw them out at once.
- Resist the temptation to use these drugs under any circumstance unless there has been a confirmed bioterrorist attack to which you have been exposed.
- Do not take medication unless you are very sure of the treatment guidelines for the specific disease you have or may have.
- Even if you have stockpiled or saved antibiotics, you should use them only after you have consulted with a doctor or medical professional knowledgeable in their specific use. Do not treat yourself.

Caretaker, Protect Thyself

After antibiotics, the most frequent purchase of those worried about bioterrorism is the gas mask. But in all but the most unusual circumstances, these expensive items are unlikely to help. Many of the gas masks sold over the Internet or in surplus shops are actually defective or expired. They may have expired air filters, cracked or brittle rubber, and many other problems and defects. Moreover, they have not been professionally sized to the individuals who would be using them—you and yours. Israel is the only country that distributes gas masks to its citizens, and there, users are individually fitted before a purchase is made. That didn't stop eight Israelis from suffocating owing to incorrect use of gas masks during the Persian Gulf War. But beyond all that, even a perfectly functional gas mask is unlikely to help. Indeed, a germ attack will most likely be covert—silent, stealthy, and accomplished hours if not days or weeks before anyone realizes it has occurred.

Gas masks are generally useless in the face of weaponized germs, but surgical masks may save your life. In fact, Dr. Rega says, you may even want to carry a simple surgical face mask around with you along with your keys and wallet. In the event you realize an attack is in progress, you could put on the mask to mitigate exposure as you attempt to vacate the epicenter of the attack.

Masks and other protective devices may turn out to be even more valuable as tools for preventing spread of contagious diease. Indeed, whether you are a physician in an emergency department, or a mother taking care of a son at home, you must use what experts call Standard Infection Control Precautions while exposed to infectious disease.

Some of the precautions are so general they apply to just about every form of infectious disease. If you are caring for anyone in a bioterrorist situation, you must wash your hands before and after you have any contact with them. If their disease is contagious, or if you fear you might be contaminated, you must wear gloves, a face shield, a cap, and a gown. Contaminated linen should be processed with chlorine bleach at high heat in your home or, possibly, discarded. You must clean and disinfect environmental surfaces and place patients at risk for contamination in a private location.

For smallpox and the viral hemorrhagic fevers, caretakers are to add to the standard precautions what physicians call "airborne" and "contact" precautions, instituted for diseases that are highly infections through touch and the air.

For airborne precautions, the patient as well as the caretaker is to wear a tight-sealing mask when being transported. Professional caretakers will often use masks with HEPA(high-efficiency particulate air) filters. But if these masks are not professionally fitted and cared for on an ongoing basis, they may not afford the intended level of protection. Nonetheless, if you are a civilian caretaker in a home situation, you will be better protected by a mask with a HEPA filter than one without it. Excellent mail order companies are recommended at the back of this book; you can even purchase a package of disposable HEPA masks at low cost. The key is getting the mask fitted by professionals, if at all possible. Do contact your local hospital to investigate how this may be done in your area.

To meet the standards of contact precautions, meanwhile, the patient must be placed in a private room. Equipment and supplies should be dedicated to one patient only, and must be cleaned and disinfected each time it is used for another patient. Further protection will be afforded by sealing the patient's room with duct tape, much like a safe room, except for areas where caretakers enter and exit.

For plague, the standard infection control precautions should be supplemented with what physicians call "droplet infection control precautions." This means the patient should be placed in a private room, and that caretakers must wear masks, goggles, and face shields when standing within 3 feet of the patient. When the patient is transported, he or she must be wearing a tight face mask as well.

Pet Plans

In the days after September 11, 2001, when residents living near the World Trade Center in New York City were evacuated from their apartments, many were told to leave their pets at home. Those who did suffered days of anxiety as animals remained trapped in boarded-up buildings, often without food. It was only when complaints hit network news that authorities forced landlords to open up buildings, and police escorted residents up through unstable structures to retrieve beloved pets before they died. Some animals, of course, did die in their isolation. Others were so traumatized that their behavior, especially their sociability, was forever changed.

To avoid this outcome with your pets, make sure that you take them with you at the time of evacuation. You should do so even if responders tell you that you will be back soon, or that the animals will be fine. There is no way to guarantee this, especially under unpredictable conditions of biological attack. Evacuating with your animals is the only way to ensure they will be fine.

Do keep in mind that Red Cross shelters don't allow pets. Therefore, you will need to find a place for your animal to board until the emergency is at an end. This is an arrangement you should make in advance, but the very uncertainty of biological attack means the animal shelter you planned on may not be available, after all. You must be prepared to seek shelter for your pet on the fly. As occurred during the World Trade Center attack in New York, you should be able to find a good Samaritan who will take your animal in temporarily, either for a fee or, as frequently occurred in New York City, free.

Remember to prepare a disaster kit for your pet, just as you have done for yourself. Items to include: medications, medical records, and a first aid kit; leashes, harnesses, or carriers so the pet cannot escape; photos of your pet, in case it gets lost; food, water, and bowls; written information on feeding schedules, medical conditions, behavior problems, and the name and number of your veterinarian in case a pet must board.

In the Aftermath: Post-Traumatic Stress

You must be prepared for the likelihood that members of your family will suffer post-traumatic stress disorder as a result of the attack. "Treatment of survivors in the acute aftermath of traumatic events is complex," according to Arieh Y. Shalev, M.D., Department of Psychiatry, Hadassah University Hospital, Jerusalem, and "survivors' concrete needs may be very urgent."

Yet just when you and your family require psychological help most, there is not a professional therapist to be found. According to the National Center for Post-Traumatic Stress Disorder, in fact, families on their own, though suffering, may have to rely on "self-help" and "self-care."

Terrorist events may affect people on all levels of involvement, whether they have merely witnessed the events or have been a direct victim. Just as other aggressive assaults waged during wartime, bioterrorism can lead to anger, frustration, helplessness, fear, and a desire for revenge. These are dangerous feelings to have when psychological help may be unavailable, or when you may be under severe duress for weeks. Do keep in mind that even under the most adverse of circumstances, the following coping strategies will help:

- Focus on brief time intervals when in a problem-solving mode (e.g., thinking only about what to do next) or focus on extended time intervals to obtain a less devastating picture of the trauma (e.g., as one tragic event in a full and meaningful life).
- Maintain a view of the self as competent and of others as willing and able to provide support.
- Focus on the current implications of the trauma and avoid regretting past decisions and actions.
- Share feelings with other survivors for support.
- Practice relaxation exercises, including deep breathing, meditation, yoga, stretching, prayer, listening to quiet music, spending time in nature, and so on.
- Participate in positive distractions: art and music, chess or a crossword puzzle will all do the trick.
- Express your feelings in a journal.

In the aftermath of an attack, experts add, self-help may include a return to the familiar, including seeing old movies and friends and rereading favorite books.

Parents must be particularly attuned to the needs of children, who may be especially prone to Post-Traumatic Stress Disorder (PTSD) in the wake of a terrorist attack. Some of the best advice comes from the National Center for Post Traumatic Stress Disorder, which notes a range of symptoms, with reactions becoming more severe the closer the child is to the terrorist event. Researchers studying the Oklahoma City bombing learned that even viewing events on TV can evoke some symptoms of PTSD.

Writing for the center, psychologist Jessica Hamblen notes that symptoms can often be classified by age. For very young children, age 6 and under, exposure to terrorism can result in feelings of helplessness and passivity on the one hand or generalized fear and heightened arousal on the other. Look here for such signs of post-traumatic stress as "freezing," marked by sudden immobility; generalized fear and heightened arousal, including an out-of-proportion startle response to loud or unusual noises. The very young may also "regress," suddenly reverting to bedwetting, demonstrating separation anxiety, and losing speech or motor skills. These very young children may also have sleep disturbances, including nightmares, as well as headaches and stomachaches caused by stress.

Starting from age 6, children may also have feelings of responsibility and guilt related to disaster. They may become preoccupied with danger, and even avoid going to school. Often, they show changes in mood, behavior and personality—either withdrawing from others or becoming aggressive and tending to angry outbursts.

Preteens and teens, meanwhile, may become suddenly rebellious or depressed. They may find it difficult to concentrate or perform well in school. The experience of trauma may cause them to act out with reckless, risk-taking behavior.

Hamblen advises: Parents must help children of all ages talk about the event and get in touch with their feelings. Honesty is important but, as the same time, so is reassurance and, to the extent possible, instilling a feeling of safety. "Provide accurate information, but make sure it is appropriate to their developmental level," Hamblen notes. "Very young children may be protected because they are not old enough to be aware that something bad has happened. School age children will need help understanding what has happened. You might want to tell them that there has been an unexpected disaster, and that many people have been hurt or killed. Adolescents will have a better idea of what has happened. Talk to them about terrorism and how the United States responds to terrorism." For older children, she adds, details are important: "Reassure children that the state and federal government, police, firemen, and hospitals are doing everything possible. Explain that people from all over the country and from other countries are offering their services."

Since children will often take on the anxiety of adults around them, it is important for parents to place the attack in perspective. "Although you yourself may be anxious or scared, children need to know that what they witnessed or heard about regarding the attack is a rare event," Hamblen advises. "Most people will never be attacked by terrorists and the world is generally a safe place."

Age Appropriate Strategies for Helping Children Cope with Traumatic Stress

Infancy to 2½:

- Maintain child's routines around sleeping and eating.
- Avoid unnecessary separations from important caretakers.
- Provide additional soothing activities.
- Maintain calm atmosphere in child's presence.
- Avoid exposing child to reminders of trauma.
- Expect child's temporary regression; don't panic.
- Help verbal child to give simple names to big feelings; talk about event in simple terms during brief chats.
- Give simple play props related to the actual trauma to a child who is trying to play out the frightening situation (a doctor's kit, a toy ambulance, and so on).

2½ to 6 Years:

- Listen to and tolerate child's retelling of event.
- Respect child's fears; give child time to cope with fears.
- Protect child from reexposure to frightening situations and re-

minders of trauma, including scary TV programs, movies, stories, and physical or locational reminders of trauma.
- Accept and help the child to name strong feelings during brief conversations (the child cannot talk about these feelings or the experience for long).
- Expect and understand child's regression while maintaining basic household rules. Expect some difficult or uncharacteristic behavior.
- Set firm limits on hurtful or scary play and behavior.
- Avoid nonessential separations from important caretakers with fearful children. Maintain household and family routines that comfort child.
- Avoid introducing new and challenging experiences for child.
- Provide additional nighttime comforts when possible: night lights, stuffed animals, physical comforting after nightmares.
- Explain to child that nightmares come from the fears a child has inside, that they aren't real, and that they will occur less and less over time.
- Provide opportunities and props for trauma-related play.
- Use detective skills to discover triggers for sudden fearfulness or regression.
- Monitor child's coping in school and day care by communication with teaching staff and expressing concern.

6 to 11 Years:

- Listen to and tolerate child's retelling of event.
- Respect child's fears; give child time to cope with fears.
- Increase monitoring and awareness of child's play, which may involve secretive reenactments of trauma with peers and siblings; set limits on scary or hurtful play. Permit child to try out new ideas to cope with fearfulness at bedtime; extra reading time, radio on, listening to a tape in the middle of the night to undo the residue of fear from a nightmare.
- Reassure the older child that feelings of fear or behaviors that feel out of control or babyish (e.g., night wetting) are normal after a frightening experience and that the child will feel more like himself or herself with time.

(continued)

Preteens and Teens:

- Encourage younger and older adolescents to talk about traumatic event with family members.
- Provide opportunities for young person to spend time with friends who are supportive and meaningful.
- Reassure young person that strong feelings—whether of guilt, shame, embarrassment, or wish for revenge—are normal following a trauma.
- Help young person find activities that offer opportunities to experience mastery, control and self-esteem.
- Encourage pleasurable physical activities such as sports and dancing.

Civilian Deputies

Should we fall victim to a bioterrorist attack of catastrophic proportion, cut off from the resources we now take for granted, each family will be only as safe as the preparation and education it has managed to amass. Under such trying circumstances, however, society as a whole will pull through most effectively when these families come together, contributing knowledge to the group and embracing teamwork to assist public health experts in delivering the appropriate information, treatment, support, and care—not just to those in the inner family circle, but to neighbors and friends.

The idea that civilians be deputized to aid first responders in their own defense was elegantly expressed this winter in *Clinical Infectious Diseases*, the prestigious journal of the Infectious Diseases Society of America. According to the authors, Thomas A. Glass of the Center on Aging and Health and Department of Epidemiology and Monica Schoch-Spana from the Center for Civilian Biodefense Studies, Johns Hopkins University Bloomberg School of Public Health, Baltimore, Maryland, "With more sophisticated awareness of the challenges posed by an epidemic caused by an act of biological terrorism, the definition of a 'first responder' to such an event is necessarily evolving." Up until now, they point out, involvement of civilians in emergency situations has been seen as an impediment. The view from the top, they note, has been that civilians may be "irrational, uncoordinated, and uncooperative in emergencies not to mention prone to panic." But the September 11, 2001, experience has shown this view to be wrong. "In New York," say Glass and Schoch-Spana, "individual volunteers and organized groups converged on the epicenter of destruction to offer aid and support, despite hazardous conditions and uncertainty about the risks of further attack or structural collapse of the World Trade Center towers. Volunteers responded rapidly and in large numbers to help in search and rescue efforts while professional operations were yet to be put in place."

In the event of a catastrophic biological attack, nothing less will be required from civilians if the thousands, if not millions, of victims are to survive. "Preparedness programs would benefit now from discussions about how to capitalize on the effectiveness and resourcefulness of nonprofessionals, especially in the identification, surveillance, and containment of an outbreak, and, potentially, in caring for large numbers of casualties," this respected journal states. "Resourceful, adaptive behavior is the rule rather than the exception in communities beset by technological and natural disasters as well as epidemics. As planning for responses to acts of bioterrorism evolves, it is important to develop strategies that enlist the public as essential and capable partners. The recent terrorist attacks in New York and Washington, D.C., draw attention to the important role of nonprofessional individuals and groups in the immediate and long-term response to disasters with mass casualties that cannot be contained within a perimeter of yellow tape. Involving the public will require, in part, raising of the general public's awareness of their roles and responsibilities after a biological attack."

Dr. Paul Rega, long experienced as a first responder on disaster scenes, notes this view must be tempered with the need to defer to expertise. "First responders in any disaster have always been the lay public," he says. "Nonetheless, we must keep in mind that while they may be saving lives, there is also a risk that they could be endangering lives—of victims, and of themselves. For instance, a nurse in Oklahoma City lost her life when a piece of masonry fell and struck her on the head. She had no protection for working at a disaster site. In a terrorist attack, an unsophisticated public could trip off a secondary explosive device and kill others accidentally." In the case of bioterrorism, civilian responders trying to help may, if inadequately prepared, expose themselves to disease. "We are not going to change human behavior," states

Dr. Rega, "but we have a duty to educate people as to the consequences of their action, and we have to let them know how they can minimize mistakes."

In the most basic sense, knowledge is power. The effort individuals and families put into educating themselves on the issue of bioterrorism and preparing for potential attacks might pay off many times over for themselves and for the communities in which they live.

RESOURCES

A. Characteristics of Biological Agents

Disease	Human transmission	Infective Dose (aerosol)	Incubation Period	Duration of Illness	Lethality (approx. case fatality rates)	Persistence of Organism	Vaccine Efficacy (aerosol exposure)
Inhalation anthrax	No	3,000–50,000 spores are theorized, but experts say it may vary widely with anthrax sample	1–6 days	3–5 days (usually fatal if untreated)	High	Very stable—spores remain viable for decades in soil	Experimental and controversial. Said to protect against anthrax, but reports of side effects disturbing.
Brucellosis	No	10–100 organisms	5–60 days (usually 1–2 months)	Weeks to months	<5% untreated	Very stable	No vaccine
Cholera	Rare	10–500 organisms	4 hours–5 days (usually 2–3 days)	≥1 week	Low with treatment, high without	Unstable in aerosols and fresh water; stable in salt water	Short-term and only 50% effective
Glanders	Low	Assumed low	10–14 days via aerosol	Death in 7–10 days in septicemic form	>50%	Very stable	No vaccine
Pneumonic plague	High	100–500 organisms	2–3 days	1–6 days (usually fatal)	High unless treated within 12–24 hours	For up to 1 year in soil; 270 days in live tissue	Vaccine not efficacious.

(continued)

Disease	Human transmission	Infective Dose (aerosol)	Incubation Period	Duration of Illness	Lethality (approx. case fatality rates)	Persistence of Organism	Vaccine Efficacy (aerosol exposure)
Tularemia	No	10–50 organisms	2–10 days (average 3–5)	2 weeks or more	Moderate if untreated	For months in moist soil or other media	80% protection
Q fever	Rare	1–10 organisms	10–40 days	2–14 days	Very low	For months on wood and sand	Experimental, and effective in guinea pigs.
Smallpox	High	Assumed low (10–100 organisms)	7–17 days (average 12)	4 weeks	High to moderate	Very stable	Vaccine protects against large doses in primates
Venezuelan equine encephalitis	Low	10–100 organisms	2–6 days	Days to weeks	Low	Relatively unstable	Experimental versions only.
Viral hemorrhagic fevers	Moderate	1–10 organisms	4–21 days	Death in 7–16 days	High for Zaire strain, moderate with Sudan	Relatively unstable—depends on agent	No vaccine
Botulism	No	Botulism is the most toxic substance on Earth; it requires 1 nanogram per kilogram of body weight to kill a human, or .7–.9 micrograms.	1–5 days	Death in 24–72 hours; lasts months if not lethal	High without respiratory support	For weeks in non-moving water and food	3-dose efficacy 100% effective in primates

Staph enterotoxin B	No	SEB is rarely lethal, but 30 nanograms can kill a person; there are 1,000 nanograms in a microgram.	3–12 hours after inhalation	Hours	Less than 1% die.	Resistant to freezing	No vaccine
Ricin	No	Lethal dose for ricin is very high. For instance, you would need 4 metric tons to kill half the people in a 100 square meter area, while you would need just a kilogram of anthrax.	18–24 hours	Days—death within 10–12 days for ingestion	High	Stable	No vaccine
T-2 mycotoxins	No	About 35 milligrams can kill 50% of those exposed.	2–4 hours	Days to months	Moderate	For years at room temperature	No vaccine

B. Cross Reference of Biological Agents

		Anthrax	Botulism	Brucellosis	Plague	Q Fever	Ricin	Smallpox	SEB	T2	Tularemia	VEE	VHF
DERMAL													
ACRAL GANGRENE	peripheral tissue death				•								
ECCHYMOSIS	bruising				•								•
ERYTHEMA	skin redness												
PAPULES	raised skin lesion							•					
PETECHIAE	pinpoint bruises				•			•					•
PURPURA	large bruising				•								•
RASH	skin eruptions			•				•			•		•
ULCERS		•									•		
VESICLES	blisters							•		•			
GASTROINTESTINAL													
ABDOMINAL PAIN		•		•	•		•	•		•			•
DIARRHEA		•		•	•		•		•				•
HEMATEMESIS	bloody vomit						•			•			•
HEMATOCHEZIA	red, bloody feces	•					•			•			•
MELENA	black, bloody stools	•								•			•
VOMITING			•	•	•	•	•	•	•	•		•	•
NEUROLOGICAL													
ATAXIA	muscular incoordination									•		•	
BLURRED VISION			•							•			
BULLAE	large blisters		•										
COMA												•	•
CONFUSION						•		•		•		•	
DELIRIUM	confusion/hallucination							•				•	•
DIPLOPIA	double vision		•			•							

		Anthrax	Botulism	Brucellosis	Plague	Q Fever	Ricin	Smallpox	SEB	T2	Tularemia	VEE	VHF
DIZZINESS			•							•			
DYSARTHRIA	difficulty speaking		•										
DYSPHAGIA	difficulty swallowing		•										
DYSPHONIA	altered voice		•										
ENCEPHALITIS	brain inflammation					•		•				•	•
HEADACHE				•	•	•		•	•		•	•	•
INTRACRANIAL HEMORRHAGE													
MENINGITIS		•		•	•							•	
MYDRIASIS	dilated pupils		•										
OBTUNDATION	mental dullness											•	
PARALYSIS			•										
PARESIS	muscle weakness		•									•	
PHOTOPHOBIA	light sensitivity		•									•	
PTOSIS	droopy eyelids		•										
SEIZURES										•		•	
RESPIRATORY													
CHEST PAIN		•		•	•	•	•		•	•	•	•	
COUGH		•		•	•	•	•		•	•	•	•	
CYANOSIS		•	•		•		•			•			
DYSPNEA		•	•		•	•	•		•	•	•		
HEMOPTYSIS	bloody sputum										•		•
PLEURAL EFFUSIONS		•									•		
PNEUMONIA					•	•			•		•		•
PULMONARY EDEMA							•			•			
STRIDOR	abnormal upper airway sound	•			•								

(continued)

SYSTEMIC		Anthrax	Botulism	Brucellosis	Plague	Q Fever	Ricin	Smallpox	SEB	T2	Tularemia	VEE	VHF
ANEMIA													
ARTHRALGIA	joint pain			•		•	•						
CHILLS		•		•	•	•		•	•		•	•	
DIC	clotting disorder	•											•
EDEMA		•											•
EPISTAXIS	nose bleed									•			•
FEVER		•		•	•	•	•	•	•		•	•	•
FLU SYMPTOMS		•		•	•	•	•	•	•		•	•	•
MALAISE	ill feeling	•	•		•	•	•	•			•		•
MYALGIA	muscle pain	•		•	•		•	•	•		•	•	•
PANCYTOPENIA	decrease of blood cells									•			
RIGORS	chills							•	•				
SHOCK		•	•		•		•			•			•
WEAKNESS			•	•			•			•		•	
WEIGHT LOSS				•		•					•		
OTHER													
ENDOCARDITIS	inner heart inflammation			•		•							
EYE PAIN							•			•	•		
HEPATIC DAMAGE					•					•	•		•
HEPATITIS				•		•							
MEDIASTINITIS	mediastinal inflammation	•											
OSTEOMYELITIS	bone infection							•					
PHARYNGITIS		•	•								•	•	
RENAL FAILURE							•				•		
SACROILIITIS	pelvic bone inflammation			•									
VERTEBRAL OSTEOMYELITIS				•									

C. Victim Instruction Form

If you fear you have been a victim of a biological attack, your first plan of action should be to interact with the official health care pipeline. By getting treatment designed by national experts for the specific agent involved, you will provide yourself and your family with the best chance of survival. To prepare for this eventuality, you might make a list of all hospitals in your area, keeping in mind that teaching and research hospitals will generally deliver the highest quality of care.

Before you set out to a hospital, you might also listen to the radio to find out if other centers have been set up. Officials may set up emergency care field tents and clinics in high schools. As large numbers of people head to the hospitals, depleting supplies of medicines and supports, you may find that the ad hoc facilities are better stocked. If you need a respirator or some antitoxin, going to a temporary facility might be the best decision yet.

You will need to decide where to go based on information from local radio stations, as well as word of mouth. Since supplies may be low, you are well advised to get what you need early in the course of events, and early in the unfolding of any disease.

Make sure that you have a copy of the following form for each member of your family, and have it filled out each time you seek treatment for a bioterrorism event. In the event of a terrorist assault, you may be confused and dazed. If you have been exposed to an agent of bioterrorism, you may be suffering neurological damage that causes brain fog, memory loss, and disorientation. You may not remember everything the doctor has instructed you to do, and as a result, you may be unable to reap the benefit of treatments or cures. To make sure you understand the instructions that have been given to you by medical professionals and other emergency workers, make copies of the form below for each family member. Do not leave an emergency room or doctor's office without the following information, in writing. You can fill in part of the form right now:

Your name:_____

Your address:_____

Contact information: Home, cell, e-mail

_____

Name of hospital, clinical, or facility where you were
seen: _____

Address of facility where you were
seen: _____

Phone number of facility were you were
seen: _____

Date and time when you were seen:_____

Names of doctors and nurses and their direct contact numbers:

_____   _____

_____   _____

I have been examined for:_____

I have received the following tests: _____

I have been diagnosed with: _____

I have been told to wait for diagnosis, and to contact the hospital
in: _____ days

I have been given no medication: _____

I have been given medication: _____

If so, note the:

Name: _____

Dose: _____

Special Instructions:

I am to take the medication for_____ days

I am to return to the clinic or hospital after _____ days

After I leave I am to (check one or more):
_____Return home
_____Resume normal activities
_____Remove all possibly contaminated clothes and secure them in
     a plastic bag
_____Shower thoroughly
_____Quarantine at home (permit entry only to immediate family)
_____Notify my doctor

I am to return to the hospital or call 911 if I experience:
_____Fever
_____Difficulty breathing
_____Difficulty speaking
_____Profound weakness
_____Flu (headache, chills, muscle aches, nausea, vomiting, diarrhea,
cough, chest pain)
_____Behavioral changes (loss of sleep, loss of appetite, inability to
function normally, emotional outbursts, irrational fears)

Other symptoms to look for (have the staff at the hospital fill this
in for you):_____
Additional instructions: _____
Doctor's signature:_____
(Ask the treating physician to sign and date this so that you have a
record of the treatment that you received.)

D. Lexicon of Biological Terror

Here are some terms you will learn as you read this volume or, alternatively, as you go beyond this handbook to read the references cited. Definitions come from *USAMRIID Medical Management of Biological Casualties Handbook,* Fort Detrick, Frederick, Md., 1998; *Stedman's Electronic Medical Dictionary,* Williams & Wilkins, Baltimore, Md., 1996; and *Principles and Practice of Infectious Diseases,* Mandell et al., 3rd ed.

Active immunization: The act of artificially stimulating the body to develop antibodies against infectious disease by the administration of vaccines or toxoids.

Analgesic: 1. A compound capable of producing analgesia, i.e., one that relieves pain by altering perception of nociceptive stimuli without producing anesthesia or loss of consciousness. 2. Characterized by reduced response to painful stimuli.

Anticonvulsant: An agent that prevents or arrests seizures.

Antitoxin: An antibody formed in response to and capable of neutralizing a biological poison; an animal serum containing antitoxins.

Anuria: Absense or defective excretion of urine.

Arthralgia: Severe pain in a joint, especially one not inflammatory in character.

Ataxia: An inability to coordinate muscle activity during voluntary movement, so that smooth movements occur. Most often due to disorders of the cerebellum or the posterior columns of the spinal cord; may involve the limbs, head, or trunk.

Bronchitis: Inflammation of the mucous membrane of the bronchial tubes.

Brucella: A genus of encapsulated, nonmotile bacteria (family Brucellaceae) containing short, rod-shaped to coccoid, gram-negative cells. These organisms are parasitic, invading all animal tissues and causing infection of the genital organs, the mammary gland, and the respiratory and intestinal tracts, and are pathogenic for man and various species of domestic animals. They do not produce gas from carbohydrates.

Bubo: Inflammatory swelling of one or more lymph nodes, usually in the groin; the confluent mass of nodes usually suppurates and drains pus.

Cerebrospinal: Relating to the brain and the spinal cord.

Chemoprophylaxis: Prevention of disease by the use of chemicals or drugs.

Cholinergic: Relating to nerve cells or fibers that employ acetylcholine as their neurotransmitter.

CNS: Abbreviation for central nervous system.

Coagulopathy: A disease affecting the coagulability of the blood.

Conjunctiva, pl. conjunctivae: The mucous membrane covering the anterior surface of the eyeball and the posterior surface of the lids.

CSF: Abbreviation for cerebrospinal fluid.

Cutaneous: Relating to the skin.

Cyanosis: Bluish discoloration of the skin suggesting lack of oxygen.

Cytotoxin: Substance that has a toxic effect on cells.

Diaphoresis: Perspiration.

Diplopia: The condition in which a single object is perceived as two objects.

Dysarthria: A disturbance of speech and language due to emotional stress, to brain injury, or to paralysis, incoordination, or spasticity of the muscles used for speaking.

Dysphagia, dysphagy: Difficulty in swallowing.

Dysphonia: Altered voice production.

Dyspnea: Shortness of breath, a subjective difficulty or distress in breathing, usually associated with disease of the heart or lungs; occurs normally during intense physical exertion or at high altitude.

Eczema: Generic term for inflammatory conditions of the skin; followed often by scaling and occasionally by hyperpigmentation; often accompanied by sensations of itching and burning.

Edema: An accumulation of an excessive amount of watery fluid in cells, tissues, or serous cavities.

Encephalitis, pl. encephalitides: Inflammation of the brain.

Endotoxemia: Presence in the blood of endotoxins.

Endotracheal intubation: Passage of a tube through the nose or mouth into the trachea for maintenance of the airway during anesthesia or for maintenance of an imperiled airway.

Enterotoxin: A cytotoxin specific for the cells of the intestinal mucosa.

Epizootic: 1. Denoting a temporal pattern of disease occurrence in an animal population in which the disease occurs with a frequency clearly in excess of the expected frequency in that population during a given time interval. 2. An outbreak (epidemic) of disease in an animal population; often with the implication that it may also affect human populations.

Erythema: Redness of the skin due to capillary dilatation.

Erythrocyte: A mature red blood cell.

Extracellular: Outside the cells.

Extraocular: Adjacent to but outside the eyeball.

Febrile: Characterized by or relating to fever.

Fomite: Objects, such as clothing, towels, and utensils that possibly harbor a disease agent and are capable of transmitting it.

Fulminant hepatitis: Severe, rapidly progressive loss of hepatic function due to viral infection or other cause of inflammatory destruction of liver tissue.

Generalized vaccinia: Secondary lesions of the skin following vaccination which may occur in subjects with previously healthy skin but are more common in the case of traumatized skin, especially in the case of eczema (eczema vaccinatum). In the latter instance, generalized vaccinia may result from mere contact with a vaccinated person. Secondary vaccinial lesions may also occur following transfer of virus from the vaccination to another site by means of the fingers (autoinoculation).

Glanders: A chronic debilitating disease of horses and other equids, as well as some members of the cat family, caused by *Burkholderia mallei*; it is transmissible to humans. It attacks the mucous membranes of the nostrils of the horse, producing an increased and vitiated secretion and discharge of mucus, and enlargement and induration of the glands of the lower jaw.

Hematemesis: Vomiting of blood.

Hyperesthesia: Abnormal acuteness of sensitivity to touch, pain, or other sensory stimuli.

Hypotension: Subnormal arterial blood pressure.

Immunoassay: Detection and assay of substances by serological (immunological) methods; in most applications the substance in question serves as antigen, both in antibody production and in measurement of antibody by the test substance.

In vitro: In an artificial environment, as in a test tube or culture media.

In vivo: In the living body.

Inoculation: Introduction into the body of the causative organism of a disease.

Microscopy: Investigation of minute objects by means of a microscope.

Moribund: Dying; at the point of death.

Myalgia: Muscular pain.

Narcosis: General and nonspecific reversible depression of neuronal excitability, produced by a number of physical and chemical agents, usually resulting in stupor rather than in anesthesia.

Necrosis: Pathologic death of one or more cells, or of a portion of tissue or organ, resulting from irreversible damage.

Nosocomial: Denoting a new disorder (not the patient's original condition) associated with being treated in a hospital, such as a hospital-acquired infection.

Oliguria: Scanty urine production.

Oropharynx: The portion of the pharynx that lies posterior to the mouth; it is continuous above with the nasopharynx via the pharyngeal isthmus and below with the laryngopharynx.

Osteomyelitis: Inflammation of the bone marrow and adjacent bone.

Pandemic: Denoting a disease affecting or attacking the population of an extensive region, country, continent; extensively epidemic.

Papule: A small, circumscribed, solid elevation on the skin.

Parasitemia: The presence of parasites in the circulating blood; used especially with reference to malarial and other protozoan forms, and microfilariae.

Passive immunity: Providing temporary protection from disease through the administration of exogenously produced antibody (i.e., transplacental transmission of antibodies to the fetus or the injection of immune globulin for specific preventive purposes).

PCR: Polymerase chain reaction.

Percutaneous: Denoting the passage of substances through unbroken skin, for example, by needle puncture, including introduction of wires and catheters.

Pharyngeal: Relating to the pharynx.

Pharyngitis: Inflammation of the mucous membrane and underlying parts of the pharynx.

Photophobia: Morbid dread and avoidance of light. Photosensitivity, or pain in the eyes with exposure to light, can be a cause.

Pleura: One of two membranes covering the lungs.

Pleurisy: Inflammation of the pleura.

Polymerase chain reaction: An in vitro method for enzymatically synthesizing and amplifying defined sequences of DNA in molecular biology. Can be used for improving DNA-based diagnostic procedures for identifying unknown biowarfare agents.

Polyuria: Excessive excretion of urine.

Prophylaxis, pl. prophylaxes: Prevention of disease or of a process that can lead to disease.

Prostration: A marked loss of strength, as in exhaustion.

Ptosis, pl. ptoses: In reference to the eyes, drooping of the eyelids.

Pulmonary edema: Edema of the lungs.

Sarin: A nerve poison that irreversibly inhibits acetylcholine, a neurotransmitter that enables nerve cells in the brain to communicate.

Sepsis: A serious infection caused by bacteria that have entered a wound or body tissue that leads to the formation of pus, or to the spread of the bacteria in the blood.

Septic shock: Shock associated with sepsis, usually associated with abdominal and pelvic infection complicating trauma or operations.

Sequela, pl. sequelae: A condition following as a consequence of a disease.

Shigellosis: Bacillary dysentery caused by bacteria of the genus *Shigella*, often occurring in epidemic patterns.

Spore: An environmentally resistant form of a microorganism, usually produced when nutritional or other outside sources of sustenance are withdrawn; capable of converting to a reproductively viable organism when resources are restored.

Superantigen: An antigen that interacts with the T cell receptor in a domain outside of the antigen recognition site. This type of interaction induces the activation of larger numbers of T cells compared to antigens that are presented in the antigen recognition site.

Superinfection: A new infection in addition to one already present.

Tachycardia: Rapid beating of the heart, usually over 100 beats per minute.

T cell: A blood cell derived from the thymus, involved in coordinating the immune system.

Teratogenicity: The property or capability of producing fetal malformation.

Toxoid: A modified bacterial toxin that has been rendered nontoxic (commonly with formaldehyde) but retains the ability to stimulate the formation of antitoxins (antibodies) and thus producing an active immunity. Examples include botulinum, tetanus, and diphtheria toxoids.

Vaccine: A suspension of attenuated live or killed microorganisms (bacteria, viruses, or rickettsiae), or fractions thereof, administered to induce immunity and thereby prevent infectious disease.

Vaccinia: An infection, primarily local and limited to the site of inoculation, induced in man by inoculation with the vaccinia (coxpox) virus in order to confer resistance to smallpox (variola). On about the third day after vaccination, papules form at the site of inoculation which become transformed into umbilicated vesicles and later pustules; they then dry up, and the scab falls off on about the 21st day, leaving a pitted scar; in some cases there are more or less marked constitutional disturbances.

Varicella: Chicken pox, an acute contagious disease, usually occurring in children, caused by the varicella-zoster virus, a member of the family Herpesviridae, and marked by a sparse eruption of papules, which become vesicles and then pustules, like that of smallpox although less severe and varying in stages, usually with mild constitutional symptoms; incubation period is about 14 to 17 days.

Variola: Smallpox.

Viremia: The presence of virus in the bloodstream.

Zoonosis: An infection or infestation shared in nature by humans and other animals that are the normal or usual host; a disease of humans acquired from an animal source.

E. Contact in Case of Emergency

Contact the following groups to obtain information or report an attack:

- National Response Center (for chem-bio hazards and terrorist events): 1-800-424-8802 or 1-202-267-2675
- National Domestic Preparedness Office (for civilian use): 1-202-324-9025
- USAMRIID Emergency Response Line: 1-888-872-7443
- CDC's Emergency Response Line: 1-770-488-7100
- Johns Hopkins Center for Civilian Biodefense Studies: 1-410-223-1667

Recommended Web Sites:

CDC Bioterrorism Preparedness and Response Program
www.bt.cdc.gov

Johns Hopkins University Center for Civilian Biodefense Studies
www.hopkins-biodefense.org

Center for Nonproliferation Studies, Monterey Institute
for International Studies
www.cns.miis.edu

Center for Terrorism Preparedness–The University of Findlay
www.ufctp.org

The Henry L. Stimson Center for Chemical and Biological Weapons Nonproliferation Project
www.stimson.org/cwc/index.html

Center for the Study of Bioterrorism and Emerging Infections—St. Louis University School of Public Health
www.slu.edu/colleges/sph/bioterrorism

FEDERAL BUREAU OF INVESTIGATION (FBI) FIELD OFFICES

FIELD OFFICE	STREET ADDRESS	ZIP CODE	TELEPHONE NO.
Albany, NY	200 McCarty Avenue	12209	(518)465-7551
Albuquerque, NM	415 Silver Avenue, SW, Suite 300	87102	(505)224-2000
Anchorage, AK	101 East 6th Avenue	99501	(907)258-5322
Atlanta, GA	2635 Century Parkway, NE; Suite 400	30345	(404)679-9000
Baltimore, MD	7142 Ambassador Road	21244	(410)265-8080
Birmingham, AL	2121 8th Avenue, N., Room 1400	35203	(205)326-6166
Boston, MA	One Center Plaza, Suite 600	02108	(617)742-5533
Buffalo, NY	One FBI Plaza	14202	(716)856-7800
Charlotte, NC	400 S. Tryon Street, Suite 900, Wachovia Blvd.	28285	(704)377-9200
Chicago, IL	219 S. Dearborn Street, Room 905	60604	(312)431-1333
Cincinnati, OH	550 Main Street, Room 9000	45202	(513)421-4310
Cleveland, OH	1240 East 9th Street, Room 3005	44199	(216)522-1400
Columbia, SC	151 Westpark Blvd.	29210	(803)551-1200
Dallas, TX	1801 N. Lamar, Suite 300	75202	(214)720-2200
Denver, CO	1961 Stout Street, Room 1823, FOB	80294	(303)629-7171
Detroit, MI	477 Michigan Avenue, P.V. McNamara FOB, 26th Floor	48226	(313)965-2323
El Paso, TX	Suite 3000, 660 South Mesa Hills Drive	79912	(915)832-5000
Honolulu, HI	300 Ala Moana Blvd., Room 4-230, Kalanianaole FOB	96850	(808)521-1411
Houston, TX	2500 East T.C. Jester	77008	(713)693-5000
Indianapolis, IN	575 N. Pennsylvania St., Room 679, FOB	46204	(317)639-3301
Jackson, MS	100 W. Capitol Street, Suite 1553, FOB	39269	(601)948-5000
Jacksonville, FL	7820 Arlington Expy., Suite 200	32211	(904)721-1211
Kansas City, MO	1300 Summit Street	64105	(816)221-6100
Knoxville, TN	710 Locust Street, Suite 600	37902	(423)544-0751

FIELD OFFICE	STREET ADDRESS	ZIP CODE	TELEPHONE NO.
Las Vegas, NV	John Lawrence Bailey Bldg., 700 E. Charleston Blvd.	89104	(702)385-1281
Little Rock, AR	10825 Financial Centre Pkwy., Suite 200	72211	(501)221-9100
Los Angeles, CA	11000 Wilshire Blvd., Suite 1700 FOB	90024	(310)477-6565
Louisville, KY	600 Martin Luther King Jr. Pl., Room 500	40202	(502)583-3941
Memphis, TN	225 North Humphreys Blvd., Suite 3000, Eagle Crest Bldg.	38120	(901)747-4300
Miami, FL	16320 NW 2nd Avenue, N. Miami Beach	33169	(305)944-9101
Milwaukee, WI	330 E. Kilbourn Avenue, Suite 600	53202	(414)276-4684
Minneapolis, MN	111 Washington Avenue South, Suite 1100	55401	(612)376-3200
Mobile, AL	One St. Louis Street, 3rd Floor, One St. Louis Centre	36602	(334)438-3674
New Haven, CT	150 Court Street, Room 535 FOB	06510	(203)777-6311
New Orleans, LA	1250 Poydras Street, Suite 2200	70113	(504)522-4671
New York City, NY	26 Federal Plaza, 23rd Floor	10278	(212)384-1000
Newark, NJ	One Gateway Center, 22nd Floor	07102	(973)622-5613
Norfolk, VA	150 Corporate Blvd.	23502	(757)455-0100
Oklahoma City, OK	50 Penn Place, Suite 1600	73118	(405)290-7770
Omaha, NE	10755 Burt Street	68114	(402)493-8688
Philadelphia, PA	600 Arch Street, 8th Floor; William J. Green, Jr., FOB	19106	(215)418-4000
Phoenix, AZ	201 E. Indianola Avenue, Suite 400	85012	(602)279-5511
Pittsburgh, PA	700 Grant Street, Suite 300 USPO	15219	(412)471-2000
Portland, OR	1500 S.W. 1st Avenue, Suite 400; Crown Plaza Bldg.	97201	(503)224-4181
Richmond, VA	111 Greencourt Road	23228	(804)261-1044
Sacramento, CA	4500 Orange Grove Avenue	95841	(916)481-9110
Salt Lake City, UT	257 East 200 South, Suite 1200	84111	(801)579-1400
San Anonio, TX	615 E. Houston Street, Suite 200; U.S. Post Office & Courthouse Building	78205	(210)225-6741
San Diego, CA	9797 Aero Drive	92123	(619)565-1255
San Francisco, CA	450 Golden Gate Avenue, 13th Floor	94102	(415)553-7400
San Juan, PR	150 Carlos Chardon, Room 526; U.S. Federal Building, Hato Roy, PR	00918	(787)754-6000
Seattle, WA	915 Second Avenue, Room 710	98174	(206)622-0460
Springfield, IL	400 W. Monroe Street, Suite 400	62704	(217)522-9675
St. Louis, MO	2222 Market Street	63103	(314)231-4324
Tampa, FL	500 E. Zack Street, Suite 610 FOB	33602	(813)273-4566
Washington, D.C.	601 4th Street, NW	20535	(202)278-2000

Directory of State and Territorial Public Health Directors

Alabama
Alabama Department of Public
Health
State Health Officer
Phone No. (334) 206-5200
Fax No. (334) 206-2008

Alaska
Division of Public Health
Alaska Department of Health and
Social Services
Director
Phone No. (907) 465-3090
Fax No. (907) 586-1877

American Samoa
Department of Health
American Samoa Government
Director
Phone No. (684) 633-4606
Fax No. (684) 633-5379

Arizona
Arizona Department of Health
Services
Director
Phone No. (602) 542-1025
Fax No. (602) 542-1062

Arkansas
Arkansas Department of Health
Director
Phone No. (501) 661-2417
Fax No. (501) 671-1450

California
California Department of Health
Services
State Health Officer

Phone No. (916) 657-1493
Fax No. (916) 657-3089

Colorado
Colorado Department of Public
Health and Environment
Executive Director
Phone No. (303) 692-2011
Fax No. (303) 691-7702

Connecticut
Connecticut Department of Public
Health
Commissioner
Phone No. (860) 509-7101
Fax No. (860) 509-7111

Delaware
Division of Public Health
Delaware Department of Health
and Social Services
Director
Phone No. (302) 739-4700
Fax No. (302) 739-6659

District of Columbia
DC Department of Health
Acting Director
Phone No. (202) 645-5556
Fax No. (202) 645-0526

Florida
Florida Department of Health
Secretary and State Health Officer
Phone No. (850) 487-2945
Fax No. (850) 487-3729

Georgia
Division of Public Health

Georgia Department of Human
Resources
Director
Phone No. (404) 657-2700
Fax No. (404) 657-2715

Guam
Department of Public Health and
Social Services
Government of Guam
Director of Health
Phone No. (67l) 735-7102
Fax No. (671) 734-5910

Hawaii
Hawaii Department of Health
Director
Phone No. (808) 586-4410
Fax No. (808) 586-4444

Idaho
Division of Health
Idaho Department of Health and
Welfare
Administrator
Phone No. (208) 334-5945
Fax No. (208) 334-6581

Illinois
Illinois Department of Public
Health
Director of Public Health
Phone No. (217) 782-4977
Fax No. (217) 782-3987

Indiana
Indiana State Department of Health
State Health Commissioner
Phone No. (317) 233-7400
Fax No. (317) 233-7387

Iowa
Iowa Department of Public Health
Director of Public Health
Phone No. (515) 281-5605
Fax No. (515) 281-4958

Kansas
Kansas Department of Health and
Environment
Director of Health
Phone No. (785) 296-1343
Fax No. (785) 296-1562

Kentucky
Kentucky Department for Public
Health
Commissioner
Phone No. (502) 564-3970
Fax No. (502) 564-6533

Louisiana
Louisiana Department of Health
and Hospitals
Asst. Secretary and State Health
Officer
Phone No. (504) 342-8093
Fax No. (504) 342-8098

Maine
Maine Bureau of Health
Maine Department of Human
Services
Director
Phone No. (207) 287-3201
Fax No. (207) 287-4631

Mariana Islands
Department of Public Health and
Environmental Services
Commonwealth of the Northern
Mariana Islands

Secretary of Health and
Environmental Services
Phone No. (670) 234-8950
Fax No. (670) 234-8930

Marshall Islands
Republic of the Marshall Islands
Majuro Hospital
Minister of Health and
Environmental Services
Phone No. (692) 625-3355
Fax No. (692) 625-3432

Maryland
Maryland Department of Health
and Mental Hygiene
Secretary
Phone No. (410) 767-6505
Fax No. (410) 767-6489

Massachusetts
Massachusetts Department of
Public Health
Commissioner
Phone No. (617) 624-5200
Fax No. (617) 624-5206

Michigan
Michigan Department of
Community Health
Chief Executive and Medical
Officer
Phone No. (517) 335-8024
Fax No. (517) 335-9476

Micronesia
Department of Health Services
FSM National Government
Secretary of Health
Phone No. (691) 320-2619
Fax No. (691) 320-5263

Minnesota
Minnesota Department of Health
Commissioner of Health
Phone No. (651) 296-8401
Fax No. (651) 215-5801

Mississippi
Mississippi State Department of
Health
State Health Officer and Chief
Executive
Phone No. (601) 960-7634
Fax No. (601) 960-7931

Missouri
Missouri Department of Health
Director
Phone No. (573) 751-6001
Fax No. (573) 751-6041

Montana
Montana Deptartment of Public
Health and Human Services
Director
Phone No. (406) 444-5622
Fax No. (406) 444-1970

Nebraska
Nebraska Health and Human
Services System
Chief Medical Officer
Phone No. (402) 471-8399
Fax No. (402) 471-9449

Nevada
Division of Health
NV State Department of Human
Resources
State Health Officer
Phone No. (702) 687-3786
Fax No. (702) 687-3859

New Hampshire
New Hampshire Department of
Health and Human Services
Medical Director
Phone No. (603) 271-4372
Fax No. (603) 271-4827

New Jersey
New Jersey Department of Health
and Senior Services
Commissioner of Health
Phone No. (609) 292-7837
Fax No. (609) 292-0053

New Mexico
New Mexico Department of Health
Secretary
Phone No. (505) 827-2613
Fax No. (505) 827-2530

New York
New York State Department of
Health
ESP-Corning Tower, 14th Floor
Albany, NY 12237
Commissioner of Health
Phone No. (518) 474-2011
Fax No. (518) 474-5450

North Carolina
North Carolina Department of
Health and Human Services
State Health Director
Phone No. (919) 733-4392
Fax No. (919) 715-4645

North Dakota
North Dakota Department of
Health
State Health Officer
Phone No. (701) 328-2372
Fax No. (701) 328-4727

Ohio
Ohio Department of Health
Director of Health
Phone No. (614) 466-2253
Fax No. (614) 644-0085

Oklahoma
Oklahoma State Department of
Health
Commissioner of Health
Phone No. (405) 271-4200
Fax No. (405) 271-3431

Oregon
Oregon Health Division
Oregon Department of Human
Resources
Administrator
Phone No. (503) 731-4000
Fax No. (503) 731-4078

Palau, Republic of
Ministry of Health, Republic of
Palau
Minister of Health
Phone No. (680) 488-2813
Fax No. (680) 488-1211

Pennsylvania
Pennsylvania Department of Health
Secretary of Health
Phone No. (717) 787-6436
Fax No. (717) 787-0191

Puerto Rico
Puerto Rico Department of Health
Secretary of Health
Phone No. (787) 274-7602
Fax No. (787) 250-6547

Rhode Island
Rhode Island Department of Health
Director of Health

Phone No. (401) 277-2231
Fax No. (401) 277-6548

South Carolina
South Carolina Department of
Health and Environmental Control
Commissioner
Phone No. (803) 734-4880
Fax No. (803) 734-4620

South Dakota
South Dakota State Department of
Health
Secretary of Health
Phone No. (605) 773-3361
Fax No. (605) 773-5683

Tennessee
Tennessee Department of Health
State Health Officer
Phone No. (615) 741-3111
Fax No. (615) 741-2491

Texas
Texas Department of Health
Commissioner of Health
Phone No. (512) 458-7375
Fax No. (512) 458-7477

Utah
Utah Department of Health
Director
Phone No. (801) 538-6111
Fax No. (801) 538-6306

Vermont
Vermont Department of Health
Commissioner
Phone No. (802) 863-7280
Fax No. (802) 865-7754

Virgin Islands
Virgin Islands Department of
Health
Commissioner of Health
Phone No. (340) 774-0117
Fax No. (340) 777-4001

Virginia
Virginia Department of Health
State Health Commissioner
Phone No. (804) 786-3561
Fax No. (804) 786-4616

Washington
Washington State Department of
Health
Acting Secretary of Health
Phone No. (360) 753-5871
Fax No. (360) 586-7424

West Virginia
Bureau for Public Health
West Virginia Department of
Health and Human Resources
Commissioner of Health
Phone No. (304) 558-2971
Fax No. (304) 558-1035

Wisconsin
Division of Health
Wisconsin Department of Health
and Family Services
Administrator
Phone No. (608) 266-1511
Fax No. (608) 267-2832

Wyoming
Wyoming Department of Health
Director
Phone No. (307) 777-7656
Fax No. (307) 777-7439

F. Decontamination, Precaution, Sanitation, Quarantine: The Supplies

Cleanliness and cautionary supplies mentioned throughout the chapters are so inexpensive and ordinary they can usually be purchased in neighborhood stores. But here are other sources, as well:

Surgical supplies, including face masks, gowns, scrubs, and gloves

AllHeart.com—Professional Appearances, Inc.
www.allheart.com/
431 Calle San Pablo
Camarillo, CA 93012
Fax: (805) 445-8816
Email Address:
customerservice@allheart.com

Buymed.com—Kern Surgical Supply
2823 Gibson St.
Bakersfield, CA 93308
Phone: (661) 327-8643
Fax: (661) 327-2730
Online Catalog: *www.buymed.com*
Sales: *buymed@buymed.com*
Customer Support:
buymed@buymed.com
Webmaster:
webmaster@buymed.com

Surgical911.com
1381 Boston Post Road
Old Saybrook, CT 06475
Voice: (800) 414-8256
Fax: (860) 395-0922
Online Catalog:
www.surgical911.com
Sales:
sales@surgical911.com
Customer Service:
service@surgical911.com
Advertising: *ads@surgical911.com*

Chief Supply Corp.
http://www.chiefsupply.com/
2468 West 11th Ave.
PO BOX 22610
Eugene, OR 97402
Phone numbers: (541) 342-4624
(800) 824-4338

Decontamination Kits, SWAT Suits, Masks for Biochemical Protection, and More

The Centech Group, Inc.
www.centechgroup.com
4600 North Fairfax Drive,
Suite 400
Arlington, Virginia 22203
Phone: (703) 525-4444
Fax: (703) 525-2349

Response Equipment Company
www.r-e-c.com
Toll Free: (888) 732-3838
Phone: (410) 671-0056
Fax: (410) 671-0058

Platinum Defense—
Israeli Gas Masks
www.platinumdefense.com
20533 Biscayne Blvd. # 4-101

Miami, FL 33180
Phone: (305) 866-9885
Fax: (305) 866-9815
info@PlatinumDefense.com

Safe Room/Negative Pressure Room
American Safe Air.com Inc.
PO BOX 2454
Mountain Home, AR 72654-2454
asa@americansafeair.com
Toll Free (888) 492 6193
or (870) 425 4405

William Lehman
Cell phone (870) 404 2510
will@americansafeair.com

Specific brands of protective equipment have been recommended by the Committee on R&D Needs for Improving Civilian Medical Response to Chemical and Biological Terrorism Incidents, Health Science Policy Program, Institute of Medicine and Board on Environmental Studies and Toxicology , Commission on Life Sciences, National Research Council.

Type	Product	Manufacturer
Breathing		
	RP51A Respirator canister	Cabot Safety Products
	PBE (Protective Breathing Equipment)	Essex PB&R Corp.
	SCU (Self-Contained Unit)	Essex PB&R Corp.
	VRU (Victim Rescue Unit)	Essex PB&R Corp.
	Plus 10 Filter Breathing Unit	Essex PB&R Corp.
	Escape hood/mask for VIPs	Fume-Free, Inc.
	QuickMask Respiratory Protective Escape Device	Fume-Free, Inc.
	FRENZY AIR 5000 breathing apparatus	Giat Industries (France)
	Respiratory protection filter kits	Giat Industries
	SPIROMATIC 90	Giat Industries
	Recirculation Filter Blower	ILC Dover, Inc.
	CAPS (Civilian Adult Protective System)	Israel Ministry of Defense Export Organization (SIBAT)
	CHIPS (Chemical Infant Protective System)	Israel Ministry of Defense Export Organization (SIBAT)
	Children Hood Blower System	Israel Ministry of Defense Export Organization (SIBAT)
	Advanced Crew Member Blower System	Israel Ministry of Defense Export Organization (SIBAT)
	Portable Blower Infant Protective Crib	Israel Ministry of Defense Export Organization (SIBAT)
	M17 series masks	MSA Defense Products
	Respirator canister Model 800375	MSA Safety Products
	ESP Mask Communication System	MSA Safety Products
	Escort (SCBA) Escape Self Contained Breathing Apparatus	Racal
	Respirator Canister Model 456-00-07R 06	Racal
	Disposable respirators	Racal
	Respirator canister Model 110100	Survivair
	M-40A1 series masks	Tradeways (Md)
	Method for filtering CB agents from airflow in confined space	TSWG (R&D only)
	First Responders mask (FIRM)	TSWG (R&D only)
Clothing		
	Mark IV permeable NBC Suit	ADI (UK)
	Remploy Tyvek F-M(ilitary) ensemble	ADI

Type	Product	Manufacturer
	JLIST (Joint Service Lightweight integrated NBC protective suit technology)	CBDCOM (R&D only)
	STEPO (Self-contained toxic environment protective outfit)	Chemfab Corp (NH)
	Biomimetic materials	DARPA/Molecular Geodesics (R&D only)
	Man-in-Simulant Test Program	Dugway Proving Grounds (R&D only)
	Low-cost protective suits	Geomet Technologies
	Field Marking Kits	Giat Industries
	TOM suit kit	Giat Industries
	Gastight suit for internal breathing apparatus	Giat Industries
	UNISCAPH gastight suit for external BA	Giat Industries
	Cool Vest Personal Cooling Garment	ILC Dover, Inc.
	Chemturion: Reusable Level A Suit	ILC Dover, Inc.
	Ready I Limited Use Level A Suit	ILC Dover, Inc.
	Cooling Vests	Kappler Protective Apparel and Fabrics
	Responder CSM Garments	Kappler Protective Apparel and Fabrics
	Pressure test kits	Kappler Protective Apparel and Fabrics
	Chemical Protective Overgarment	Marine Corps Systems Command (R&D only)
	Functionally Tailored Fibers and Fabrics	Natick RDEC (R&D only)
	Firefighters Integrated Protective Suit—Combat (FISC)	Natick RDEC (R&D only)
	Advanced Lightweight Chemical Protection	Natick RDEC (R&D only)
	Level B Suit	Responder-Geomet
	Level A Suit	Responder-Geomet
	SARATOGA-Pyjama Chemical Protective Undergarment	Tex-Shield, Inc (NJ)
	CW-66 Chemical Protective Flight Coverall	U.S. Air Force
	(BDO) Battledress overgarment	Winfield International (NY)
Clothing and Breathing		
	Domestic Preparedness Civilian PPE Testing Program	CBDCOM (R&D only)
	(CBPSS) Chemical Biological Protective Shelter System	Engineered Air Systems (MO)
	Individiual Protective Kit	Giat Industries
	Rescue and Lifting Kit	Giat Industries
	Ventilated casualty bag	Giat Industries

Type	Product	Manufacturer
	Ventilated casualty hood	Giat Industries
	ILC Dover Transportable Collective Protection System	ILC Dover
	M20A1 SCPE (Simplified Collective Protection System)	ILC Dover, Inc.
	Improvements to existing C/B Bomb suit	Tech Escort Unit (R&D only)
	Expedient Hazard Reduction System	TSWG (R&D only)
	ILC Dover Transportable Collective Protection System	ILC Dover
	Protection assessment test system	U.S. Army (R&D only)

Decontamination Equipment Recommended by the Committee on R&D Needs for Improving Civilian Medical Response to Chemical and Biological Terrorism Incidents, Health Science Policy Program, Institute of Medicine and Board on Environmental Studies and Toxicology, Commission on Life Sciences, National Research Council.

Product	Source/Location
M11, M13 Man-portable decontamination application systems	All-Bann Enterprises/Tradeways Ltd (MD)
M12 Powered vehicle-mounted multipurpose decontaminating apparatus	All-Bann Enterprises/Tradeways Ltd (MD)
DS2P Decon solution	All-Bann Enterprises/Tradeways Ltd (MD)
M17 Lightweight decontamination system (Sanator)	Engineered Air Systems (MO)
Emergency Response Equipment Package	HAZ/MAT DQE Inc (IN)
Hospital-based Decontamination Equipment Package	HAZ/MAT DQE Inc (IN)
Transportable Decontamination Systems	Modec Inc. (Denver)
Decontamination Kit No. 2	Tradeways Ltd
M291 Decontamination kit for individual equipment	Tradeways Ltd
M258 Skin decontamination kit	Tradeways Ltd

G. Medications and Therapies

Please note: You must obtain all your medical prescriptions from licensed and trained physicians, and through the health care pipeline that will be set up in case of an emergency. You should defer to these physicians and experts on all medications that you take. In the event of a catastrophic biological strike by terrorists, however, experts' scenarios predict that the health care pipeline may shut down. In this instance, you may be forced to go further than the corner drugstore to obtain the medication your doctor wants you to take.

Following is a list of legitimate Internet pharmacies you can access should your local drugstores or hospitals be short on medication or simply unavailable:

- Drugstore.com: *www.drugstore.com*
- PlanetRx: *www.planetrx.com*
- Rite Aid: *www.riteaid.com*
- Rx.com: *www.rx.com*
- Soma.com: *www.soma.com*
- Walgreens: *www.walgreens.com*
- Yourpharmacy: *www.yourpharmacy.com*

Antibiotic Supplies for Pets

Just as you defer to medical doctors in treating you and your family, so, too, should you defer to veterinarians in treating your pets. But in the case of a catastrophe, you are far less likely to find a vet than an M.D. Indeed, while the government will do all it can to rapidly set up medical services for humans, the same emergency services for cats and dogs will probably be rare to absent. Yet your pets can contract the same diseases causing havoc for you.

For pets, the online venue of choice is Drs FosterSmith, a well-known and highly reputable catalog company. The company sells a full line of pet products, including antibiotics available only by prescription from a veterinarian. In addition, the company sells nonprescription antibiotics for fish, including penicillin, ampicillin, tetracycline, amoxicillin, cephalexin, metronidazole, and erythromycin.

You must never treat pets with antibiotics, let alone antibiotics intended for an alternate species, without the express instructions of your veterinarian. However, in a catastrophic situation, your veterinarian may be unable to get a written prescription out. Under such circumstances, you may be able to acquire only the nonprescription drugs. If that is the case, use medications for one species to treat another *only* if you have specific instructions from a veterinary expert acting as guide.

Drs FosterSmith:
www.drsfostersmith.com
(800) 381-7179
Doctors Foster & Smith
P.O. Box 100
Rhinelander, WI 54501-0100

If you have birds, you can obtain prescription and nonprescription antibiotics for them through Back Street Birds, located in Scottsdale, Arizona, at *www.backstreetbirds.com*.

Respiratory Resources

Helping a loved one survive biological attack may sometimes mean providing adequate ventilation. These days, most of us would never think of providing ventilation without a stay at the hospital and then subsequent employment of a trained home health care aide or respiratory therapist. But in the event of a national catastrophe, your hospital may have no remaining beds for patients in need, and approval of insurance companies as well as official involvement of home health care companies may be difficult to secure. You may need to fend for yourself in terms of finding equipment and help, and you may do so, in part, through the listings below:

Organizations That Can Help with Respiratory Needs

Note: It may be difficult to impossible to line up sophisticated respiratory help in your home in the wake of a catastrophic bioterrorism attack. The best way to obtain such support is through a public health care pipeline that has been established to deliver this level of care. Should official response be slow in coming, you can try to call the following organizations for advice.

The ALS Association (ALSA)
27001 Agoura Road, Suite 150
Calabasas Hills, CA 91301-5104
800-782-4747
818-880-9007
818-880-9006 fax
alsinfo@alsa-national.org
www.alsa.org

American Association for
Respiratory Care (AARC)
11030 Ables Lane
Dallas, TX 75229-4524
972-243-2272
972-484-2720 fax
info@aarc.org
www.aarc.org

American College of Chest
Physicians (ACCP)
3300 Dundee Road
Northbrook, IL 60062-2348

847-498-1400
847-498-5460 fax
accp@chestnet.org
www.chestnet.org

American Sleep Apnea Association
1424 K St. NW, Suite 302
Washington, DC 20005
202-293-3650
202-293-3656 fax
www.sleepapnea.org

American Syringomyelia Alliance
Project
PO Box 1586
Longview, TX 75606-1586
800-272-7282
903-236-7079
903-757-7456 fax
pwilliams13@compuserve.com
www.syringo.org
www.asap4sm.com

American Thoracic Society (ATS)
1740 Broadway
New York, NY 10019-4374
212-315-8700
212-315-6498 fax
info@lungusa.org
www.thoracic.org

CCHS Family Network
71 Maple Street
Oneonta, NY 13820-1561
607-432-8872
607-431-4351 fax
VanderlaanM@hartwick.edu
www.cchsnetwork.org

Charcot-Marie-Tooth Association
(CMTA)
2700 Chestnut Street
Chester, PA 19103-4867
800-606-2682
610-499-9264
610-499-9267 fax
cmtassoc@aol.com
www.charcot-marie-tooth.org

Christopher Reeve Paralysis
Foundation (CRPF)
500 Morris Avenue
Springfield, NJ 07081
800-225-0292
973-912-9433 fax
paralysis@aol.com
www.paralysis.org

Communication Independence for
Neurologically Impaired, Inc.
(CINI)
116 John Street, Suite 1304
New York, NY 10038-3301
212-385-8045

212-385-9724 fax
cini@cini.org
www.cini.org

Concepts of Independence, Inc.
Consumer Directed Personal
Assistance Program
120 Wall Street, Suite 1010
New York, NY 10005
212-293-9999
212-293-3040 fax
conceptscdpa@earthlink.net
www.conceptscdpap.org

Cystic Fibrosis Foundation
6931 Arlington Road
Bethesda, MD 20814
800-344-4823
301-951-4422
301-951-6378 fax
info@cff.org
www.cff.org

Disability Information and
Resources
PO Box 82433
Kenmore, WA 98028-0433
jlubin@eskimo.com
www.eskimo.com/~jlubin/disabled/
vent/index.html

Families of SMA (Spinal Muscular
Atrophy)
PO Box 196
Libertyville, IL 60048-0196
800-886-1762
847-367-7620
847-367-7623 fax
sma@fsma.org
www.fsma.org

Families of SMA of Louisiana
3350 Ridgelake Drive, Suite 150
Metairie, LA 70002
504-828-0010
504-828-0899 fax

Family Support Network
1850 E. 17th Street, Suite 104
Santa Ana, CA 92705-8625
714-543-7600

Family Voices
PO Box 769
Algodones, NM 87001
888-835-5669
505-867-2368
505-867-6517 fax
kidshealth@familyvoices.org
www.familyvoices.org

FSH (Facioscapulohumeral)
Society Inc.
3 Westwood Road
Lexington, MA 02420
781-860-0501
781-860-0599 fax
carol.perez@fshsociety.org
www.fshsociety.org

Guillain Barré Syndrome
Foundation International
PO Box 262
Wynnewood, PA 19096
610-667-0131
610-667-7036 fax
gbint@ix.netcom.com
www.webmast.com/gbs/

Independence Crossroads, Inc.
8932 Old Cedar Avenue South
Bloomington, MN 55425

952-854-8004
952-854-7842 fax
info@independencecrossroads.org
www.independencecrossroads.org

Independent Living Research
Utilization (ILRU)
Research and Training Ctr
2323 S. Shepherd Drive, Suite 1000
Houston, TX 77019
713-520-0232
713-520-5136 TTY
713-520-5785 fax
www.ilru.org

Les Turner ALS Foundation Ltd.
8142 Lawndale
Skokie, IL 60076
847-679-3311
847-679-9109 fax
info@lesturnerals.org
www.lesturnerals.org

Muscular Dystrophy Association
(MDA)
3300 E. Sunrise Drive
Tucson, AZ 85718-3208
800-572-1717
520-529-5300 fax
mda@mdausa.org
www.mdausa.org

Myasthenia Gravis Foundation
123 W. Madison Street, Suite 800
Chicago, IL 60602-4503
800-541-5454
312-853-0522
312-853-0523 fax
myastheniagravis@msn.com
www.myasthenia.org

National Association for Medical Direction of Respiratory Care (NAMDRC)
5454 Wisconsin Avenue, Suite 1270
Chevy Chase, MD 20815
310-718-2975
301-718-2976 fax
namdrc@erols.com
www.namdrc.org

National Association for Ventilator-Dependent Individuals (NAVDI)
11607 Euclid Avenue, Apt. 303
Cleveland, OH 44106
216-791-6362
swilpula@aol.com

National Association of Pediatric Home and Community Care
UMass Memorial Healthcare
Department of Pediatrics
55 Lake Avenue N. Rm S5-860
Worcester, MA 01655
508-856-1908
508-856-2609 fax
dorothy.page@banyan.ummed.edu

National Coalition to Amend the Homebound Restriction
13831 Hutchings Court
Watsonville, CA 95076
831-728-7764
831-728-5123 fax
NCAHB1@aol.com
www.amendhomeboundpolicy.home stead.com

National Information Center for Children and Youth with Disabilities (NICHCY)
PO Box 1492

Washington, DC 20013-1492
800-695-0285
202-884-8200 tel/TTY
202-884-8441 fax
nichcy@aed.org
www.nichcy.org

National Organization for Rare Disorders, Inc. (NORD)
PO Box 8923
New Fairfield, CT 06812-8923
203-746-6518
203-746-8728 fax
orphan@rarediseases.org
www.rarediseases.org

National SCI Hotline
2200 Kernan Drive
Baltimore, MD 21207
800-526-3456
410-448-6627 fax
scihotline@aol.com
www.scihotline.org

The National Scoliosis Foundation
5 Cabot Place
Stoughton, MA 02072-4624
800-673-6922
781-341-6333
781-341-8333 fax
scoliosis@aol.com
www.scoliosis.org

National Spinal Cord Injury Association (NSCIA)
8701 Georgia Avenue, Suite 500
Silver Spring, MD 20910-3723
800-962-9629
301-588-9414 fax
resource@spinalcord.org
www.spinalcord.org

Paralyzed Veterans of America
(PVA)
801 18th Street NW
Washington, DC 20006-3715
800-872-8200
202-872-1300
800-795-4327 TDD
www.pva.org

The Parent Project for Muscular
Dystrophy Research, Inc.
1012 N. University Blvd.
Middletown, OH 45042
800-714-KIDS
513-424-0696
513-425-9907 fax
www.parentdmd.org

Pierre Robin Network
PO Box 3274
Quincy, IL 62305
217-224-7480
217-224-0292 fax
www.pierrerobin.org

Polio Survivors Association
12720 LaReina Avenue
Downey, CA 90242
562-862-4508
562-862-5018 fax
www.polio-association.org

Respiratory Nursing Society (RNS)
c/o NYSNA
11 Cornell Road
Latham, NY 12110
518-782-9400 ext 286
518-782-9530 fax (attn: Lynda
Degen)
rns@nysna.org

Respiratory Resources, Inc.
850 Amsterdam Avenue, Suite 9A
New York, NY 10025
212-666-2210
212-666-0642 fax
breethezy@aol.com

Scoliosis Association, Inc.
PO Box 811705
Boca Raton, FL 33481-1705
800-800-0669
561-994-4435
561-994-2455 fax
scoliosisassn@aol.com
www.scoliosis-assoc.org

Sick Kids (Need) Involved People
SKIP of New York, Inc.
213 W. 35th Street, 11th Floor
New York, NY 10001
212-268-5999
212 268 7667 fax

REFERENCES

Chapter 1, Anthrax

Alibek, K. Statement before U.S. Congress, 20 October 1999. Can be accessed at *www.house.gov/hasc/testimony/106thcongress/99–10–20alibek.htm.*

Armstrong, D., and J. Cohen. *Infectious Diseases.* London: Harcourt Publishers, Ltd; 1999: 8.15.8–9.

Bartlett, J.G., J. Ticehurst, and J. Zenilman, et al. *Clinical Anthrax: Primer for Physicians.* Johns Hopkins Center for Civilian Biodefense Studies; 2001. Can be seen at: *www.hopkins-biodefense.org/pages/agents/anthraxprimer111401.html.*

Brachman, P. "Inhalation anthrax." *Ann NY Acad Sci,* 1980;353:83–93.

CDC recommendation. "Update: Investigation of Bioterrorism-Related Anthrax and Interim Guidelines for Exposure Management and Antimicrobial Therapy." 26 October, *MMWR* 2001;50:909. *www.cdc.gov/mmwr/preview/mmwrhtml/mm5042a1.htm.*

Centers for Disease Control and Prevention. Transcript for program "CDC Responds: An Update on Treatment Options for Postal and Other Workers Exposed to Anthrax," videotaped 27 December 2001, at the Centers for Disease Control and Prevention, Atlanta. *www.bt.cdc.gov/DocumentsApp/Anthrax/12212001/ postalworkers update.pdf.*

Center for the Study of Bioterrorism and Emerging Infections, St. Louis University School of Public Health, Bioterrorism Agent Fact Sheet, Anthrax.

Cherry, N., et al. "Health and Exposures of United Kingdom Gulf War Veterans." Part II: The relation of health to exposure. *Occup Environ Med* 2001;58:299–306.

Dirck, J.H. "Virgil on anthrax." *AM J Dermatopathol.* 1981;3:191–195.

Dixon, T., M. Meselson, J. Guillemin and P. Hanna. "Anthrax." *N Engl J Med* 1999;341:815–826.

Franz, D.R., P.B. Jahrling, and A.M. Friedlander, et al. "Clinical recognition and management of patients exposed to biological warfare agents." *JAMA.* 1997; 278(5):399–411.

Friedlander, A.M. *Textbook of Military Medicine: Medical Aspects of Chemical and Biological Warfare.* Office of the Surgeon General Department of the Army, United States of America; 1997:467–475.

Friedlander, A.M., S.L. Welkos, and M.L. Pitt, et al. "Postexposure Prophylaxis Against Experimental Inhalation Anthrax." *Journal of Infectious Disease.* May 1993;167(5):1239–43.

Friedlander, A.M., et al. "Anthrax Vaccine: Evidence for Safety and Efficacy Against Inhalational Anthrax." *JAMA* 282;22:2104–6.

Gugliotta, G. "Anthrax Has Inspired Dread and Breakthroughs." *Washington Post,* 5 November 2001; A09.

Hayes, S.C., and M.J. World. "Adverse Reactions to Anthrax Immunization in the Military Field Hospital." *JR Army Med Corps* 2000; 146:191–5.

Institute of Medicine Committee on Health Effects Associated with Exposures During the Gulf War. Gulf War and Health Volume I: Depleted Uranium, Pyridostigmine Bromide, Sarin, Vaccines. *National Academy Press* 2000; Washington, D.C.

Jernigan, J.A., D.S. Stephens and D.A. Ashford, et al. "Bioterrorism-related Inhalational Anthrax: The First 10 Cases Reported in the United States." *Emerg Infect Dis.* 2001;7:933–944.

Koch, R. "Die Aetiologie der Milzbrand-Krankheit, begründet auf die Entwicklungsgeschichte des *Bacillus anthracis* [in German]." *Beiträge zur Biologie der Pflanzen.* 1876;2:277–310.

LaForce, F.M. "Woolsorters' Disease in England." *Bull NY Acad Med.* 1978;54:956–963.

Leggiadro, R.J. "The Threat of Biological Terrorism: A Public Health and Infection Control Reality." *Infect Control Hosp Epidemiol.* 2000; 21(1):53–56.

Malone, J.D. *Bioterrorism Readiness Audioconference.* APIC, 1999. *Medical Management of Biological Casualties Handbook.* Frederick, MD: U.S. Army Medical Research Institute of Infectious Diseases, Fort Detrick; 1999.

Meselson, M., J. Guillemin and M. Hugh-Jones, et al. "The Sverdlovsk Anthrax Outbreak of 1979." *Science* 1994;266:1202–1208.

Moran, G.J. "Biological Terrorism. Part 1: Are We Prepared?" *Emerg Med.* 2000;14–38.

Nass, M. Interview with author, December 2001 and January 2002.

Osterholm, M.T., and J. Schwartz. *Living Terrors: What America Needs to Know to Survive the Coming Bioterrorist Catastrophe.* New York, NY: Delacorte Press; 2000.

Pasteur, Chamberland, Roux. "Compte rendu sommaire des expériences faites à Pouilly-'le-Fort, près Melun, sur la vaccination charbonneuse [in French]." *Comptes Rendus des séances De L'Académie des Sciences.* 1881;92:1378–1383.

Rega, P. *Bio-Terry: A Stat Manual to Identify and Treat Diseases of Biological Terrorism.* Maumee, Ohio: MASCAP, Inc.; 2001.

"B anthracis Can Develop Resistance to Quinolones and Macroslides." *Reuters Medical News.* 18 December 2001.

Rosenbaum, D.E., and S.G. Stolberg. "U.S. Will Offer Anthrax Shots for Thousands." *New York Times,* 19 December 2001.

Rosenbaum, D.E. and S.G. Stolberg. "As U.S. Offers Anthrax Shots, Safety Debate Begins Again." *New York Times,* 20 December 2001.

Steele, L. "Prevalence and Patterns of Gulf War Illness in Kansas Veterans: Association of symptoms with Characteristics of Person, Place and Time of Military Service." *Am J Epidemiol* 2000; 152:991–1001.

Suffin, J., W. Carnes, and A. Kaufmann. "Inhalation Anthrax in a Home Craftsman." *Clinical Infectious Diseases,* 1998;26: 97–102.

Unwin, C., et al. "Health of UK Servicemen Who Served in the Persian Gulf War." *The Lancet* 1999;353:169–178.

Virgil. *The Georgics.* L.P. Wilkinson (Trans.). New York: Penguin Classics; 1983. The Georgics also available on the Internet Classics Archive at *http://classics.mit.edu/Virgil/georgics.html.*

Chapter 2, Plague

Barry, J. "Planning a Plague?" *Newsweek*. 1 February 1993:40–41.

Cavanaugh, D.C., F.C. Cadigan, J.E. Williams, and J.D. Marshall. "Plague." In: Ognibene AJ, Barrett O'N. *General Medicine and Infectious Diseases*. Vol 2. In: Ognibene AJ, Barrett O'N. *Internal Medicine in Vietnam*. Washinton, D.C.: Office of the Surgeon General and Center of Military History; 1982: Chap 8, Sec 1.

Center for the Study of Bioterrorism and Emerging Infections, St. Louis University School of Public Health. *Bioterrorism Agent Fact Sheet, Plague*.

Evans, M.E., and A.M. Friedlander. "The plague." In: *Textbook of Military Medicine: Medical Aspects of Chemical and Biological Warfare*. Office of the Surgeon General, Department of the Army. Washington, D.C.; 1997.

Inglesby, T.V., D.T. Dennis, and D.A. Henderson, et al. "Plague as a Biological Weapon: Medical and Public Health Management." *JAMA*. 2000; 283:2281–2290.

Mee, C. "How a Mysterious Disease Laid Low Europe's Masses." *Smithsonian*. 1990;20(Feb):66–79.

Rega, P. *Bio-Terry: A Stat Manual to Identify and Treat Diseases of Biological Terrorism*. Maumee, OH: MASCAP Inc.; 2001.

Williams, P., and D. Wallace. *Unit 731: Japan's Secret Biological Warfare in World War II*. New York, NY: The Free Press; 1989.

Chapter 3, Tularemia

Center for the Study of Bioterrorism and Emerging Infections, St. Louis University School of Public Health. *Bioterrorism Agent Fact Sheet, Tularemia*. www.slu.edu/colleges/sph/bioterrorism/quick/tularemia01. PDF.

Centers for Disease Control and Prevention, Public Health Emergency Preparedness and Response, Brucellosis, www.bt.cdc.gov/Agent/Tularemia/Tularemia.asp.

Dennis, D.T., et al. Working Group on Civilian Biodefense. "Tularemia As a Biological Weapon: Medical and Public Health Management." *JAMA*. 2001;285(21):2763–2773.

Evans, M.E., and A.M. Friedlander. "Tularemia." In: *Textbook of Military Medicine: Medical Aspects of Chemical and Biological Warfare*.

Office of the Surgeon General, Department of the Army. Washington, D.C.; 1997.

Medical Management of Biological Casualties Handbook, 4th ed. Frederick, MD: U.S. Army Medical Reseach Institute of Infectious Diseases, Fort Detrick; 2001.

Rega, P. *Bio-Terry: A Stat Manual to Identify and Treat Diseases of Biological Terrorism.* Maumee, OH: MASCAP Inc.; 2001.

Chapter 4, Cholera

Center for the Study of Bioterrorism and Emerging Infections, St. Louis University School of Public Health. *Bioterrorism Agent Fact Sheet, Cholera.* Available at: *www.slu.edu/colleges/sph/bioterrorism/quick/cholera01.pdf.*

Chin, J. *Control of Communicable Diseases Manual,* 17th ed., American Public Health Association, Washington, D.C.; 2000.

Finkelstein, R.A. "Cholera, Vibrio Cholerae and Other Pathogenic Vibrios" in Baron, S., Medical Microbilogy, University of Texas Medical Branch, Galveston, TX. 1996. Available at *http://gsbs.utmb.edu/microbook/ch024.htm.*

Grafstein, E., and G. Innes. "Bioterrorism: An Emerging Threat." *Canad J Emerg Med.* Vol. 1, No 3, October 1999. Available at: *www.caep.ca/004.cjem-jcmu/004-00.cjem/vol-1. 1999/v13205.htm.*

Kortepeter, M., G. Christopher, and T. Cieslak, et al. *Medical Management of Biological Casualties Handbook.* U.S. Army Medical Research Institute of Infectious Diseases, U.S. Department of Defense, February 2001.

Sidell, F.R., E.T. Takafuji, and D.R. Franz. *Military Aspects of Chemical and Biological Warfare.* Office of the Surgeon General, U.S. Army. Borden Inst., WRAMC, 1997.

Chapter 5, Q Fever

Center for the Study of Bioterrorism and Emerging Infections, St. Louis University School of Public Health. *Bioterrorism Agent Fact Sheet, Tularemia. www.slu.edu/colleges/sph/bioterrorism/quick/qfever01. PDF.*

Evans, M.E., and A.M. Friedlander. "Q fever." In: *Textbook of Military Medicine: Medical Aspects of Chemical and Biological Warfare.*

Office of the Surgeon General, Department of the Army. Washington, D.C.; 1997.

Medical Management of Biological Casualties Handbook, 4th ed. Frederick, MD: U.S. Army Medical Reseach Institute of Infectious Diseases, Fort Detrick; 2001.

Rega, P. *Bio-Terry: A Stat Manual to Identify and Treat Diseases of Biological Terrorism.* Maumee, OH: MASCAP Inc.; 2001.

Smith, R.J. "Russia Fails to Detail Germ Arms." *Washington Post.* 3 August 1992;A-1.

Chapter 6, Brucellosis

Center for the Study of Bioterrorism and Emerging Infections, St. Louis University School of Public Health. *Bioterrorism Agent Fact Sheet, Brucellosis.* www.slu.edu/colleges/sph/bioterrorism/quick/brucellae01. PDF.

Centers for Disease Control and Prevention, Public Health Emergency Preparedness and Response, Brucellosis, www.bt.cdc.gov/Agent/Brucellosis/Brucellosis.asp.

Hoover, D.L., and A.M. Friedlander. "Brucellosis." In: *Textbook of Military Medicine: Medical Aspects of Chemical and Biological Warfare.* 1997.

Medical Management of Biological Casualties Handbook, 4th ed. Frederick, MD: U.S. Army Medical Reseach Institute of Infectious Diseases, Fort Detrick; 2001.

Rega, P. *Bio-Terry: A Stat Manual to Identify and Treat Diseases of Biological Terrorism.* Maumee, OH: MASCAP, Inc.; 2001.

Young, D.A.B. "Florence Nightingale's Fever." *Brit Med J.* 1995 (23–30 Dec); 311:1697–1700.

Chapter 7, Glanders and Melioidosis

Center for the Study of Bioterrorism and Emerging Infections, St. Louis University School of Public Health. *Bioterrorism Agent Fact Sheet, Glanders.* www.slu.edu/colleges/sph/bioterrorism/quick/glanders01.PDF.

Medical Management of Biological Casualties Handbook, 4th ed. Frederick, MD: U.S. Army Medical Reseach Institute of Infectious Diseases, Fort Detrick; 2001.

Chapter 8, Smallpox

de Clercq, E., A. Holy, and I. Rosenberg. "Efficacy of Phosphonyl-methoxyalkyl Derivatives of Adenine in Experimental Herpes Simplex Virus and Vaccinia Virus Infections in Vivo. *Antimicrob Agents Chemother.* 1989; 33(2):185–191.

Franz, D.R., P.B. Jahrling, and A.M. Friedlander, et al. "Clinical Recognition and Management of Patients Exposed to Biological Warfare Agents. *JAMA.* 1997;278(5):399–411.

Henderson, D.A., T.V. Inglesby, and J.G. Bartlett, et al. "Smallpox as a Biological Weapon: Medical and Public Health Management." *JAMA.* 1999; 281:2127–2137.

Henderson, D.A., and F. Fenner. "Recent Events and Observations Pertaining to Smallpox Virus Destruction in 2002." *Clin Infec Dis.* 2001;33:1057–1059.

Kempe, C.H., C. Bowles, and G. Meiklejohn, et al. "The Use of Vaccinia Hyperimmune Gamma-globulin in the Prophylaxis of Smallpox." *Bull WHO.* 1961;25:41–48.

Koplan, J.P., K.A. Monsur, and S.O. Foster, et al. "Treatment of Variola Major with Adenine Arabinoside." *J Infect Dis.* 1975;131(1):34–39.

Leggiadro, R.J. "The Threat of Biological Terrorism: A Public Health and Infection Control Reality. *Infect Control Hosp Epidemiol.* 2000;21(1): 53–56.

McClain, D.J. *Textbook of Military Medicine: Medical Aspects of Chemical and Biological Warfare.* Office of the Surgeon General Department of the Army, Washington, D.C.; 1997: p. 539–553.

Medical Management of Biological Casualties Handbook. Frederick, MD: U.S. Army Medical Research Institute of Infectious Diseases, Fort Detrick; 1999.

Monsur, K.A., M.S. Hossain, and F. Huq, et al. "Treatment of Variola Major with Cytosine Arabinoside." *J Infect Dis.* 1975;131(1):40–43.

Moran, G.J. "Biological Terrorism. Part 1: Are We Prepared? *Emerg Med.* Feb 2000:14–38.

Osterholm, M.T., and J. Schwartz. "Living Terrors: What America Needs to Know to Survive the Coming Bioterrorist Catastrophe." New York, NY: Delacorte Press 2000.

Shuto, S., T. Obara, and M. Toriya, et al. "New Neplanocin Analogues, I: Synthesis of 6'-modified neplanocin A Derivatives as Broad-spectrum Antiviral Agents." *J Med Chem.* 1992;35(2):324–331.

Sodeik, B., G. Griffiths, and M. Ericsson, et al. "Assembly of Vaccinia Virus: Effects of Rifampin on the Intracellular Distribution of Viral Protein." *J Virol.*1994;68(2):1103–1114.

Tseng, C.K., V.E. Marquez, and R.W. Fuller, et al. "Synthesis of 3-deazaneplanocin Λ, a Powerful Inhibitor of S-adenosylhomocysteine Hydrolase with Potent and Selective in Vitro and in Vivo Antiviral Activities." *J Med Chem.* 1989;32(7):1442–1446.

Connolly, C. "HHS Set to Order Smallpox Vaccine for All Americans." *Washington Post,* 7 November 2001; A09.

CDC Interim Smallpox Response Plan and Guidelines. Draft 2.0; 11/21/01. Accessible at *www.bt.cdc.gov/DocumentsApp/Smallpox/RPG/index.asp.*

Rotz, L.D., D.A. Dotson, I.K. Damon, and J.A. Becher. Vaccinia (Smallpox) Vaccine Recommendations of the Advisory Committee on Immunization Practices (ACIP), 22 June 2001 / 50(RR10);1–25.

Chapter 9, The Viral Hemorrhagic Fevers

Alibek, K. "Behind the Mask: Biological Warfare." *Perspective.* 1998 (Sept-Oct);9(1).

Canonico, P.G., M. Kende, B.J. Luscri, and J.W. Huggins. "In-vivo Activity of Antivirals Against Exotic RNA Viral Infections." *J Antimicrob Chemother.* 1984;14(suppl A):27–41.

Centers for Disease Control Guideline. "Management of Patients with Suspected Viral Hemorrhagic Fever." *MMWR.* 1988;37[S-3]:1–16.

Centers for Disease Control and Prevention and World Health Organization. *Infection Control for Viral Hemorrhagic Fevers in the African Health Care Setting.* Atlanta, GA: Centers for Disease Control and Prevention; 1998:1–198.

Centers for Disease Control. "Management of Patients with Suspected Viral Hemorrhagic Fever." *MMWR.* 1988;37(suppl 3):1–16.

Dyer, N. "Killers Without Cures." *Science World,* 2 October 2000; 57(3):8.

Guba, W.W. "Uganda in Terror as Ebola Spreads." *London Times.* 22 October 2000.

Huggins, J.W. "Prospects for Treatment of Viral Hemorrhagic Fevers with Ribavirin, a Broad-spectrum Antiviral Drug." *Rev Infect Dis.*1989;11(4):S750–S761.

Inglesby, T.V. "The Germs of War: How Biological Weapons Could

Threaten Civilian Populations." *Washington Post,* 9 December 1998, L Edition. p. H01

Jahrling, P.B. "Viral Hemorrhagic Fevers." In: *Textbook of Military Medicine: Medical Aspects of Chemical and Biological Warfare.* Office of the Surgeon General, U.S. Department of the Army; 1997.

McCarthy, M. "A Century of the US Army Yellow Fever Research." *Lancet,* 2 June 2001; 357 (Issue 9270): 1772.

McCormick, J.B., I.J. King, and P.A. Webb, et al. "Lassa Fever: Effective Therapy with Ribavirin." *N Engl J Med.* 1986;314:20–26.

Medical Management of Biological Casualties Handbook, 4th ed. Frederick, MD: U.S. Army Medical Reseach Institute of Infectious Diseases, Fort Detrick; 2001.

Miller, J., S. Engelber, and W. Broad. *Germs.* New York: Simon & Schuster; 2001.

Nathan, N., M. Barry, M. Van Herp, and H. Zeller. "Shortage of Vaccines During a Yellow Fever Outbreak in Guinea." *Lancet* 2001; 358: 2129–30.

Rega, P. *Bio-Terry: A Stat Manual to Identify and Treat Diseases of Biological Terrorism.* Maumee, OH: MASCAP Inc; 2001.

Chapter 10, The Equine Encephalitides

Alibek, K. "Behind the Mask: Biological Warfare." *Perspective.* 1998 (Sept-Oct); 9(1).

Medical Management of Biological Casualties Handbook, 4th ed. Frederick, MD: U.S. Army Medical Reseach Institute of Infectious Diseases, Fort Detrick; 2001.

Peters, C.J., and J.M. Dalrymple. "Alphaviruses." In: Fields, B.M., and Knipe D.M., (eds.) *Virology,* 2nd ed. Vol 1. New York: Raven Press; 1990:713–761.

Rega, P. *Bio-Terry: A Stat Manual to Identify and Treat Diseases of Biological Terrorism.* Maumee, OH: MASCAP Inc.; 2001.

Smith, J.F., K. Davis, M.K. Hart, G.V. Ludwig, D.J. McClaim, M.D. Parker, W.D. Pratt. "Viral encephalitides." In: *Textbook of Military Medicine: Medical Aspects of Chemical and Biological Warfare.* Office of the Surgeon General, U.S. Department of the Army; 1997.

Strauss, J.H., and E.G. Strauss. "The Alphaviruses: Gene Expression, Replication, and Evolution." *Microbiol Rev.* 1994;58(3):491–562.

Chapter 11, Botulism

Alibek, K., S. Handleman. *Biohazard.* New York, NY: Random House; 1999.

APIC/CDC Bioterrorism Readiness Plan: A Template for Healthcare Facilities *www.apic.org/educ/readinow.html*

Arnon, S.S., R. Schechter, T. V. Inglesby, et al. "Botulinum Toxin as a Biological Weapon." *JAMA.* 2001; 285 (8):1059–1070.

Biological and Chemical Terrorism: Strategic Plan for Preparedness and Response—Recommendations of the CDC Strategic Planning Working Group *ftp://ftp.cdc.gov/pub/Publications/mmwr/RR/RR4904.pdf*

Medical Management of Biological Casualties Handbook. Frederick, MD: U.S. Army Medical Research Institute of Infectious Diseases, Fort Detrick; 1999.

Middlebrook, J.L., D.R. Franz. *Textbook of Military Medicine: Medical Aspects of Chemical and Biological Warfare.* Office of the Surgeon General, U.S. Department of the Army; 1997: 643–654.

Smithson, A.E. *Toxic Archipelago: Preventing Proliferation from the Former Soviet Chemical and Biological Weapons Complexes.* Washington, D.C.: The Henry L. Stimson Center; December 1999:7–21. Report No. 32. Available at: *www.stimson.org/cwc/toxic.htm.*

United States Department of State. *Patterns of Global Terrorism 1999.* Washington, D.C.: U.S. Dept of State; April 2000. Department of State publication 10687. Available at: *www.state.gov/www/global/terrorism/1999report/1999index.html.*

United Nations Security Council. *Tenth Report of the Executive Chairman of the Special Commission Established by the Secretary-General Pursuant to Paragraph 9(b)(I) of Security Council Resolution 687 (1991), and Paragraph 3 of Resolution 699 (1991) on the Activities of the Special Commission.* New York, NY: United Nations Security Council; 1995. S/1995/1038.

Zilinskas, R.A. "Iraq's Biological Weapons: The Past as Future?" *JAMA.* 1997;278:418–424.

Chapter 12, Yellow Rain (T-2 Mycotoxin)

Ciegler, A. "Mycotoxins: Occurrence, Chemistry, Biological Activity." *Lloydia.* 1975;38(1):21–35.

Ciegler, A., and J.W. Bennett. "Mycotoxins and Mycotoxicoses." *Bioscience.* 1980;30(8):512–515.

Joffe, A.Z. "Alimentary Toxic Aleukia." In: Kadis S, Ciegler A, Ajl SJ, eds. *Microbiological Toxins*. Vol 7. In: *Algal and Fungal Toxins*. New York, NY: Academic Press; 1971:139–189.

Medical Management of Biological Casualties Handbook, 4th ed. February Frederick, MD: U.S. Army Medical Reseach Institute of Infectious Diseases, Fort Detrick; 2001.

Rega, P. *Bio-Terry: A Stat Manual to Identify and Treat Diseases of Biological Terrorism*. Maumee, OH: MASCAP Inc.; 2001.

Wannemacher, J.R., and S.L. Weiner. "Trichothecene Mycotoxins." In: *Textbook of Military Medicine: Medical Aspects of Chemical and Biological Warfare,* Office of the Surgeon General, U.S. Department of the Army; 1997.

Yagen, B., A.Z. Joffe, and P. Horn. "Toxins From a Strain Involved in ATA." In: *Mycotoxins in Human and Animal Health,* eds, J.V. Rodericks, C.W., Hesseltine, and M.A. Mchlman. Park Forest South, Illinois: Pathotox Publishers. pp. 329–336.

Chapter 13, Staphlococcal Enterotoxin B

Medical Management of Biological Casualties Handbook, 4th ed. Frederick, MD: U.S. Army Medical Reseach Institute of Infectious Diseases, Fort Detrick; 2001.

Rega, P. *Bio-Terry: A Stat Manual to Identify and Treat Diseases of Biological Terrorism*. Maumee, OH: MASCAP Inc.; 2001.

Ulrich, R.G., S. Sidell, and T.J. Taylor. "Staphylococcal Enterotoxin B and Related Pyogenic Toxins. In: *Textbook of Military Medicine*: *Medical Aspects of Chemical and Biological Warfare,* Office of the Surgeon General, U.S. Department of the Army; 1997;3:621–631.

Chapter 14, Ricin

Carus, W.S. *Bioterrorism and Biocrimes: The Illicit Use of Biological Agents Since 1900*. Center for Counterproliferation Research, National Defense University in Washington, D.C., February 2001. Can be seen at *www.ndu.edu/centercounter/Full_Doc.pdf.*

Cookson, J., and J. Nottingham. *A Survey of Chemical and Biological Warfare*. New York, NY: Monthly Review Press; 1969:6.

Crompton, R., D. Gall, and G. Markov. "Death in a Pellet." *Med Leg J.* 1980;48:51–62.

Franz, D.R., and N.K. Jaax. "Ricin Toxin." In: *Textbook of Military Medicine: Medical Aspects of Chemical and Biological Warfare.* Office of the Surgeon General, U.S. Department of the Army; 1997.

Lloyd, A. "Bin Laden's Poison Manual." *Times* London: 16 November 2001.

Medical Management of Biological Casualties Handbook, 4th ed. Frederick, MD: U.S. Army Medical Reseach Institute of Infectious Diseases, Fort Detrick; 2001.

Rauber, A., and J. Heard. "Castor Bean Toxicity Re-examined: A New Perspective." *Hum Toxicol.* 1985;27:498–502.

Rega, P. *Bio-Terry: A Stat Manual to Identify and Treat Diseases of Biological Terrorism.* Maumee, OH: MASCAP Inc.; 2001.

Conclusion, Family Preparedness

Glass, T.A., and M. Schoch-Spana. Bioterrorism and the people: How to vaccinate a city against panic. *Clin Infect Dis.* 2002 Jan 15;34(2): 217–223.

"Family Disaster Plan." Developed by the *Federal Emergency Management Agency* and the *American Red Cross.* Copyright © 2001 The American National Red Cross. All Rights Reserved.

The Humane Society of the United States *www.hsus.org.* More information about pets from The American Veterinary Medical Association *www.avma.org/vmat/disasterbrochure.asp.*

Rega, P. *Bio-Terry: A Stat Manual to Identify and Treat Diseases of Biological Terrorism.* Maumee, OH: MASCAP Inc.; 2001.